Monster Lies

Monster Lies

A Woman's Guide to Controlling Her
Destiny

*Sally Franz
& Jennifer Webb*

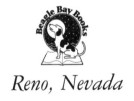

Reno, Nevada

Monster Lies
A Woman's Guide to Controlling Her Destiny

Beagle Bay Books,
a division of Beagle Bay, Inc.
Reno, Nevada
info@beaglebay.com
Visit our website at: http://www.beaglebay.com

Cover Design: Blackletter Creative
Editing Services: Vicki Hessel Werkley

Library of Congress Cataloging-in-Publication Data

Franz, Sally, 1951-
Monster lies : a woman's guide to controlling her destiny / by Sally Franz & Jennifer Webb.-- 1st trade ed.
p. cm.
ISBN 0-9679591-6-0 (alk. paper)
1. Women--Psychology. 2. Self-actualization (Psychology) 3. Self-perception in women. 4. Self-help techniques. I. Webb, Jennifer, 1947- II. Title.
HQ1206 .F695 2002
646.7'0082--dc21   2002004418

First Trade Edition
Printed in Canada

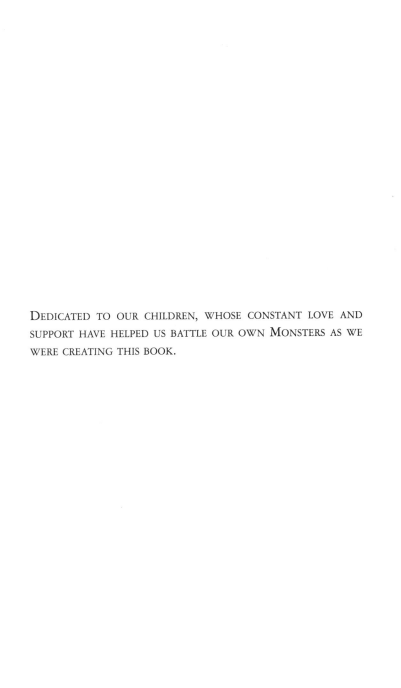

DEDICATED TO OUR CHILDREN, WHOSE CONSTANT LOVE AND
SUPPORT HAVE HELPED US BATTLE OUR OWN MONSTERS AS WE
WERE CREATING THIS BOOK.

ACKNOWLEDGEMENTS

Jennifer: Thanks to my oldest friend Linda Bloodworth-Thomason (we've known each other since first grade), whose encouragement and enthusiasm about our first draft inspired us to keep on writing, and to the winds of fate that put Jacqueline and Robin Simonds (our publishers) at the same party, so we could meet, as well as their optimism, candor and strength in helping create a stronger, more powerful book. Also thanks to our awesome editor, Vicki Werkley. Finally thanks to those dear friends who saw only light at the end our editorial tunnel, and to my-reason-for-being-on-this-planet-in-the-first-place, my family. Their unconditional love and support helped me find and keep my focus and voice: my daughter Marlo, my son Michael, my grandchildren Rachel and Sandon, my daughter-in-law Joy, my son-in-law Sean and my spoiled, deaf, soul-mate cocker spaniel, Shakespeare.

Sally: Thank you to Mark Victor Hansen for his kind words supporting *Monster Lies* and for his spirit of generosity and business savvy. Thanks to our publishers Jacqueline and Robin Simonds who had the enthusiasm and foresight to see the potential of this book. Thank you to my mother, Judith Dolezal who taught me to get up and take responsibility for my life even when I didn't feel like it. Special thanks to my twin brother Dan and sisters Janet, Carol and Sharon who made growing up an adventure. And to my children Rachel and Rebekah who let me grow up all over again with them. And over all of it I must acknowledge Jesus Christ, my personal savior who has sustained me through trial and trouble and not a small amount of my own stubborn willfulness.

Contents

Monster Lies
A Woman's Guide to Controlling Her Destiny

FOREWORD

I confess right up front that I'm a fan of *Monster Lies: A Woman's Guide to Controlling Her Destiny*. But I must also disclose that one of the authors of this extremely candid and original book is my friend, Jennifer Webb, with whom I shared a rich and rip-roaring girlhood in Southern Missouri. We have kept in touch and cared about one another through the years. Like any good friend, I knew of Jennifer's numerous struggles and triumphs, but I did not really grasp the significance of her personal experiences as they relate to the lives of so many other women. Until I read *Monster Lies*.

In a publishing market that is currently flooded with slender, gimmicky tomes on every problem known to womankind, I found *Monster Lies* refreshing with its incisive, cut-to-the-chase analysis of the many ways we as women trip ourselves up—how we not only settle for less, but in fact come to believe that less is all we deserve.

These authors, Jennifer Webb and Sally Franz, know whereof they speak. They are women who have lost everything. Several times. Both endured parental loss at an early age, unhappy and abusive marriages, overwhelming financial problems, temporary loss of their children and seemingly no dearth of people lining up to tell them that their situations were hopeless (ah, will we ever stop underestimating the female species?). Jennifer and Sally have not only beaten the odds by turning their own impossible lives into success stories, they have seen with astonishing clarity the mistakes they made and the simple truths that are available to every woman who wants another chance at genuine self-fulfillment.

The result of their new-found understanding is this very direct, no-holds-barred workbook for women of all ages. I use the term work because there are lots of places in the book where the reader can interact with the authors' ideas. One also gets to luxuriate in the often-funny female camaraderie of the writers as well as their in-your-face honesty. *Monster Lies* hits so close to home, you might feel that these ladies have tapped your phone. Every woman who reads it will discover that she has been a victim of at least one *Monster Lie* and most of us have been held hostage at one time or another by all of them. The good news about Jennifer and Sally is that they did not become successful and then leave no forwarding address. Instead, they have decided to share their blueprint for self-realization and happiness with the rest of us. At the very least, this book will leave you wanting to have lunch with them. Even better, it will change your life forever.

Linda Bloodworth-Thomason
creator of the hit TV series
Designing Women and *Evening Shade*.

Monster Lies

A Woman's Guide to Controlling Her
Destiny

INTRODUCTION

"I used to allow criticism from others to unseat me and cause me to doubt myself. Then I learned that these people were revealing more about themselves than they were about me. They just didn't know it. Now I listen and learn, and I don't confuse their views with the truth about me."

— Catherine Ryan Hyde
author of the New York Times best-seller
Pay It Forward

Are you tired of self-help books that promise you the world, but seem short on reality? You know, the ones that promise you a quick fix to all your problems, immediate solutions to everything from finding a new job to finding a new husband; from handling a serious illness to overcoming depression? The one-day diet? Let's face it, we're all looking for experts to fix whatever isn't working and to create change in our lives. So why is this book different? It's a book written by two women who have changed their lives not by trying harder, but by understanding where change comes from. Our formula is easy. If we want extraordinary RESULTS, we have to do two things:

> **REVEAL** *the* Monster Lies *that haunt us, exposing the secrets people seem afraid to talk about.*
> **ACT** *immediately to change the negative influence of these Lies.*

This book offers you all the information you need to create extraordinary results in your life. You don't have to wait two years and work ten hours a day to see these results. You can begin experiencing change immediately.

Hello, we're Sally Franz and Jennifer Webb. We met five years ago and started talking, as women are apt to do. We found out that we had parallel lives of suffering and pain, and also of success. We decided right then and there to write a book to help other women avoid the pitfalls we had experienced. We wanted to warn women of all ages of the things we'd discovered that could block their success in life. We wanted to tell you our stories and how we learned to overcome incredible odds.

First of all, we want you to know there's nothing special about us. We didn't inherit tons of money or have husbands who put us into business or have IQs high enough to dazzle corporate executives. We sure didn't have the right contacts. In fact, we pretty much lost everything we had due to the wrong contacts and other circumstances. We lost what we had more than once. In early childhood, we both experienced the pain from the loss of a parent: Jennifer's mother died when she was ten; Sally's father abandoned the family when she was two. We both married when very young—Jennifer was only seventeen, Sally twenty—and we were so destroyed emotionally by unhappy marriages and financial problems that we temporarily gave up custody of our children. Both of us then struggled to find ways to get our families back together. We were smart, ambitious and positive, yet we couldn't seem to break the cycle of pain, poverty and poor relationships. Any of this sound familiar?

Then something amazing happened to us. We became aware that somewhere, somehow, there were lots of choices out there that nobody had told us about. There were choices from how to deal with a collection agency to how to get free training and education. The key to making better choices was to start making choices that would help us take care of ourselves and our children. That was very difficult. We were so used to being bullied and compromised we barely knew how to stand up for ourselves. In fact, standing up for ourselves felt selfish and wrong.

Do you find it hard to say *no* to people who ask favors, even though it's a huge imposition? Do you over-extend yourself and then resent the people you help? That's how we felt all the time. We had to learn to put ourselves on the top of the priority list. We had to learn how to exercise our muscles of self-control. Not control that inhibits, but control to take charge of our lives, our time and our resources. We had to stop being afraid of that word *control*. We had to think of control as being responsible, not manipulative. We had to dare to start thinking about what we wanted and what our children needed, then find ways to get it. But how? We were meek and scared and could barely ask a waitress to take back spoiled food or even use a telephone without feeling self-conscious.

We now know we were not alone. Millions of women suffer from depression and low self-esteem because they believe wrongly they have no right or power over their futures. They believe they have nothing to contribute to the world, even if they could control their futures. They believe they're not special. Why else would we be seeing a steady increase of women on anti-depressant medication? Feeling lost and powerless is very real. So it's time to take back the control of your life. There are many ways to do that, but the key is to start with small baby steps first.

Introduction Exercise 1

It may seem silly, but try this small lesson in change. Prove to yourself that you have control over your life. How? Have something unpredictable for breakfast. Open up a can of vegetable soup and eat it with a pickle, etc. List here what would be the most outrageous things you could have for breakfast:

1. _____

2. _____

Now think of three things you can do to express yourself that don't cost money, but are a clear choice—no matter how small—you can make during the course of your day. Examples: Wear only one earring all day; move your office chair in a different place for the day; eat your lunch with chopsticks, even if it's a BLT on white toast; or get up ten minutes earlier and start reading a novel.

1. _____

2. _____

3. _____

If this seems way too foolish, ask yourself, "Who told me this is foolish?" You see, we've often been told that people in control are just born leaders. That's not necessarily true. Leaders and successful people learn as children how to take control of little things. Then they build up to big things. First, take control over little things to exercise your decision-making muscle. Then you can work up to running a company, running for office, running a 10K or choosing a wonderful life for yourself. We began creating change for ourselves by identifying the erroneous beliefs—or *Monster Lies*—that held us down for years, almost destroying us in the process. We talked about what Monsters we had to tame in order to move away from negativity, poverty and despair. We formed a partnership designed to shorten the learning curve of others who may be on the same journey, or perhaps are just getting ready to get on the road. You may be a housewife, a teenager, a corporate executive or a grandmother. Wherever you are in life, if you're searching for a way to break the cycle, then you need to fight back the *Monster Lies* that trap you, discourage you and rob you of your hope and energy. Each of us has had to deal with our own personal set of Lies and family secrets. We're not psychologists and cannot give you advice on your personal experiences. What we can do is identify *Monster Lies* common to us all—especially women—and tell you how we've tamed them, and how you can do the same.

CHAPTER ONE

Who Are These Monsters, Anyway?
Introducing the Monster Lies

"Why should anybody hire me?"
"I don't have the money. I'm trapped."
"I don't have a degree, so I'm never going to get anywhere."
"I'm stuck in this marriage for at least fifteen more years.
    It's hopeless."
"All my education is getting me nowhere. There's nothing
    more I can do."

The negative voices in your head are vicious liars, so harmful, unkind and destructive that we call them Monsters. In fact, the more you can see these Lies as actual Monsters (and not the Truth), the easier it will be for you to fight them off. We have identified more than seventy-five *Monster Lies* just between the two of us, but for this book we'll start off with the twelve biggest and most dangerous Lies. These are the negative beliefs that kept us from happiness and success for so many years. If you're in emotional pain, there's more than likely a *Monster Lie* somewhere close by. See if you relate to any of these. List when you've heard them and who in your life sends you these negative messages. It's crucial to know what you're telling yourself, and who's reinforcing these beliefs, in order for you to identify the Monsters and move forward.

The Twelve Monster Lies Survey

Doomsday: This Monster fills you with gloom and hopelessness about the future. "Nothing ever changes, so what's the use?"

I have heard this voice when:
Example: I got a speeding ticket
The people who talk this way:
Example: my mom.

When you conquer Doomsday you'll be able to put life's issues into perspective and regain your hope quickly.

Stressor: This Monster wants you to believe outside forces stress you out. This allows you to blame others, even though you choose the life, job and relationships you have. Stressor wants you to believe you can't do anything about all the demands on your life.

I have heard this voice when:
The people who talk this way:

When you conquer Stressor, you'll be able to quickly return to your center (be in control) and find the inner peace and strength to move forward.

Perfecto: This Monster warns that you should be an expert the very first time you try anything. "Learning curves are for wimps." Mistakes make you feel stupid and inadequate. Perfecto wants you to go through life feeling like a failure for being human. "If you can't be perfect the first time, give it up."

I have heard this voice when:

_____

The people who talk this way:

_____

When you conquer Perfecto, you'll be able to take necessary risks and be willing to make the mistakes needed in your learning curve, in order to have what you want.

Scarcity: This Monster is always afraid there won't be enough. It wants you to horde things, be stingy and be jealous of others. "Sure you have money today, but what about tomorrow?" You can never enjoy what you have because you live in fear.

I have heard this voice when:

_____

The people who talk this way:

_____

When you conquer Scarcity, your fears will be replaced with a generous and grateful heart, which is the key to prosperity. Then you'll know how to get the resources you need.

Satisfaction: Sounds like a nice pal—but wait. Satisfaction pretends It's satisfied. Satisfaction never asks for things It wants. No one ever knows It has needs. Satisfaction is waiting to be asked. "It's not polite to ask for things." Fear of rejection stops Satisfaction in Its tracks, so It settles for less and less and becomes sadder and sadder. Do you feel as if you're intruding on others if you ask?

I have heard this voice when:

The people who talk this way:

When you conquer Satisfaction, you'll learn how to ask for what you need and get it. You will feel entitled to all the resources available to you.

Experteaser: This Know-It-All thinks everyone should listen to It. "Who do you think you are?" "Who told you that you were special?" Experteaser wants you never to trust your own judgment but always to listen to others, especially people who seem smarter or are in positions of power. This way you'll probably never make a decision to change your life.

I have heard this voice when:

The people who talk this way:

When you conquer Experteaser, you'll know that no one else

is an expert on your future. You'll be able to design your own destiny with excitement and enthusiasm. You'll have confidence to know that you, and you alone, are the expert of your own life. Only you have control of your choices and your choices design the future.

Yardstick: This Monster makes you believe you must always measure up to other people's expectations. If others think you should be in business and you've always loved music, give up your dreams to please them. "Everybody knows the only real jobs, people and lifestyle that count are . . . ." Yardstick wants you to focus so hard on other people's standards that you don't even know what you like anymore.

I have heard this voice when:

_____

The people who talk this way:

_____

When you conquer Yardstick, you'll stop spending energy keeping up appearances and you'll focus on the most important person to influence: yourself. You'll make better choices because they will be in line with your own goals, not the goals of others. You'll decide what is truly important.

Stuck-in-the-Mud: This charming Monster wants you to be so busy helping other people who are stuck that you never have a life of your own. It wants you to wait until everybody else changes before you change. "How can I go back to college before my husband stops drinking?" "You don't understand, I can't write with a sick mother to take care of."

I have heard this voice when:

_____

The people who talk this way:

_____

When you conquer Stuck-in-the-Mud, you'll start investing in your own future and stop being held back by other people's issues. You see, it's so much easier to put your energy into fixing someone else's life, leaving you no time to work on your own. You'll learn to set boundaries and take care of yourself. Then you'll have the energy and resources to help others in a way that doesn't detract from your own growth.

Clairvoyant: This Monster wants you to live in the land of wishful/magical thinking. It wants you to expect that if people really liked you they could read your mind. "If you don't know why I'm upset, I'm certainly not going to tell you." "If you really loved me, you'd know what I want for my birthday."

I have heard this voice when:

_____

The people who talk this way:

_____

When you conquer Clairvoyant, you'll understand how to communicate and how to listen to others. You'll stop expecting people to know what you need without your asking. You'll learn the power of direct communication.

13

Assumption: This Monster already knows everything about other people, even people it's never met. "Oh, those people from that country—they all act that way." "I know you; you're always late." "She's too old to start over."

I have heard this voice when:

_____

The people who talk this way:

_____

When you conquer Assumption, you'll give up preconceived ideas about the world, and you'll see with new eyes. The good news: with your new beliefs, your world will have all the resources you need for the future you want.

Sandman: "Sweet dreams" is the biggest part of Sandman's Lie. This Monster wants you to go to sleep on your life. "Poor baby, why not just accept your life, be realistic, stop trying. Settle for the life you have." Maybe you think you need something for all that pain: some alcohol, drugs, sex, food, more work, or anything to make you forget. Just do something to dull the pain and go to "sleep-sleep-sleep-sleep, my pretty."

I have heard this voice when:

_____

The people who talk this way:

_____

When you conquer Sandman, you'll have the courage to face your fears head on. You'll be willing to be conscious and aware so you can live life to the fullest.

Worrywart: This Monster is an investment in a future you probably don't want anyway! Sitting around upset, confused and powerless is an interesting way to deal with things. In fact, if Worrywart has Its way, you could spend your life worrying about things that never happen. "What if something horrible happens?" Yes, but what if, instead, you live a lovely life and die of old age in your sleep at a hundred and four? Worry is a strange replacement for planning, training and coping.

I have heard this voice when:

_____

The people who talk this way:

_____

When you conquer Worrywart, you'll learn how to replace worry with action. You'll use your worry energy to create new solutions.

These _Monster Lies_ are your enemies. They're cheaters and liars that will distort the information. For instance, if somebody breaks up with you, your Monster will tell you that you're hopeless and unlovable, based on a belief that lovable people are never left. This is not true. Lovable people are left all the time—look at the divorce rates. It just feels as if we're unlovable under certain circumstances, such as when we're lonely. When we feel vulnerable, the _Monster Lies_ seem the most real to us and do the most damage, often telling us we'll never change, so why even bother trying!

Remember these important facts:

☞Monster Lies *never die.*

The sources that *Monster Lies* come from are many: superstitions, common knowledge, traditions, class systems, corporate ladders, hearsay, gossip and customs, to name a few. These are a part of civilization, creating voices that are heard everywhere. As soon as you think you've told one to shut up and buzz off, another one shows up to upset you, if not in your own head, then in the voices of others.

☞Monster Lies *are the voices of conformity.*

Many of these Lies were created to keep us within certain behavior limits, certain boundaries, as in, "Who do you think you are?" "Forget it, you'd never understand it!" and "If people were meant to fly, they'd have wings; you can't invent wings for people!" It's upsetting to the rule-makers and -keepers if you go off "half-cocked" making up new rules. If you succeed in having a new and better life, it makes a very loud statement that they were wrong. People don't like to be wrong; most will do anything to avoid being wrong. The *Monster Lies* that try to control you exist to keep you from showing up others. If you understand that, it will be easier to know exactly what you're fighting.

☞*Do not embrace the* Monster Lies.

See them for what they are. Now, some psychologists will tell you these voices are a part of you, a part you must reconcile. But we've discovered that these Monsters are body invaders. They come from the outside to poison us. In essence, they're the cultural, family and media myths that can actually ruin your life.

☞*Count on the* Monster Lies *to haunt you.*

The fact that *Monster Lies* will revisit you has nothing to do with your ability to be strong. This is not about doing enough interpersonal work. It's about the nature of the Monsters. If they sniff out a weak moment, they'll raise their ugly heads and pay you an unwelcome visit. Sometimes they even come in disguise: your Aunt Mabel, the checkout girl at Safeway, or a scrap of paper that falls from an old photo album.

Our motto is: If you feel bad, sad or scared, be on your guard for a *Monster Lie*.

When we started to write this book, we suffered through every single one of these *Monster Lies* all over again! Like some cosmic joke, if Sally was writing about Scarcity (not having enough), she would lose an entire month's worth of work. If Jennifer was writing about being afraid of making a mistake, she would humiliate herself publicly in some very special way. When Sally wrote about Doomsday, her fiancé broke off the relationship without so much as a conversation about what went wrong. If Jennifer was recreating a scenario from Stressor, she would "accidentally" bring on a very stressful event. Or she would get a visit from her special demon, Perfecto who would tell her: "Everything you do must be done perfectly, or not at all." If she felt she'd conquered something that had been especially challenging, and was happy just learning a skill, someone would inform her that she had a glaring misspelling on a handout. These are big and little traumas. Monsters like to show up when we're learning new tasks,

17

learning patience, or in the middle of a dilemma searching for the solution. They're so predictable we can now spot and handle them much sooner. Another good reason we call these voices *Monsters* is in order to recognize them. Sometimes these voices and cultural messages are so strong, or so subtle, we forget to confront them. Remember, you can fight the enemy much easier if you can recognize it!

Monster Lie Exercises

Here are the steps you can take to fight back your *Monster Lies:*

1. List all the things you're trying to accomplish (potty training a two-year-old, learning a new computer system, balancing your checkbook, creating a better résumé, breaking off a relationship, losing weight, learning a new language, relocating, etc.):

_____

_____

2. List how you feel when it doesn't go right the first time (Perfecto):

_____

_____

3. List what that means about you—what kind of a person fails? (Yardstick) What names do you use to describe someone who gets things wrong?

_____

_____

4. Do you want to give up? What else could you do to waste time and not get this job done: (Straighten house / office / garage, make a phone call, check e-mail)? (Sandman):

_____

_____

5. Who could help you? Why are you afraid to ask them for help? (Satisfaction)

_____

_____

Here's how you fight these *Monster Lies:*

You counteract Lies with the Truth. Say these slogans out loud until you believe them:

1. Everyone feels foolish doing a new task. There is no shame in asking for help.

2. No one is perfect except God. Stop trying to be God. Remember that almost every "overnight success" worked at it for ten to twenty years and made lots of mistakes along the way.

3. Many people want to help you—your job is to find them. If you're shy asking friends or coworkers, then start with librarians. They're paid to help you get information.

4. Trying to "look good" uses more energy you could spend learning. Admitting your mistakes

quickly is the sign of superior intelligence. Accomplished people know the sooner you admit what doesn't work, the closer you are to finding a solution.

That's it. Speak and act the Truth and the *Monster Lies* go away. Concentrate on where you're going, not where you've been. Look for your own unique purpose in life.

Easy idea and hard to do. Why? Because we're so heavily programmed to focus on negativity in our world. Bad news seems to travel faster than the speed of light. Good news seems boring. Of course, there really is a lot more good news than bad. Many more people have succeeded than failed. People who've had more obstacles than you face have made it, but you don't know who they are yet.

Your first assignment is to research successful people. Read biographies. For example: most of us have heard of Mrs. Fields, the woman who started a little cookie business in 1977, with her company today grossing more than $300 million from more than 1000 outlets. But when she started, there were all sorts of Monsters at her door. Even though family, friends, bankers—and her husband—said *no,* she managed to get a loan. Her husband then predicted she wouldn't sell $50 worth of cookies in her first day of business. As hours passed, there were no sales. Deciding yet again not to buy into the negative, she took a tray of cookies outside to offer samples to passers-by. At the end of the day, she'd sold $75 worth of cookies. There's one woman who refused to let the Monsters get in her way!

The other reason it's hard to speak the Truth is that sometimes we've never heard it before. So many people tell us smart people never fail, never make mistakes, never ask questions and never ask for help. Yet we never thought to ask, "OK, give us five examples." Or if we did, we were smacked or told to be quiet or to show some respect. But you're an adult now; you're a free agent. You have the right to question every bad and negative *Monster Lie* out there. It's time to go into *Monster Lie* combat training.

This is a powerful art. Learning to combat your particular *Monster Lies* will take some practice. There are exercises and reminders throughout this book to help you learn new choices. These will help you practice new thinking and actions that will enable you to achieve the life you want now. Build your muscles a little every day. Soon you'll be strong enough to face any Monster and arm-wrestle It to the ground.

We can't promise you life's problems and heartaches won't happen. Once you know about these *Monster Lies,* however, you'll be better able to fight them off and get on with your life. You can figure out what's stopping your growth, your dreams and your happiness.

How? By equipping yourself with the tools you need to recognize when you're being sabotaged by a *Monster Lie*. We can teach you how to find out the Truth about what is possible for your life. We'll show you how to practice the exercises, which will help you access your creative right-brain skills and these skills will help you accelerate your growth and truly think smarter and more quickly!

Ask yourself this: What if I really can have what I want? What if other people with even fewer skills than I possess, have conquered these barriers? What if there's a way to be happier? Pretty scary and pretty exciting, right? Do you believe you're capable of taking control of your life? Let's find out . . . .

CHAPTER TWO

Can People Really Ever Change?

When do people change? How do they break the cycle of confusion, endless frustration or pain? When they switch from talk to action—and just about any little action will do. It's an amazing thing, but once you begin to change, you build momentum. You actually get better at change as you experience success. In fact, you can learn to change any part of your life if you're willing to practice it daily. This book is all about learning to change your beliefs and actions so you can have the life you want.

When is it time to change? When you become aware of dissatisfaction in your life. What causes people to examine how they got caught up in their present situation? Often a word from a friend—not always a kind word either—a book you read, a speaker you heard. It begins when it occurs to you there may be hope for a better life. It begins when you believe there is a better way. It is the first ray of hope.

Sally

"I'm so angry with Bert!" the voice on the phone blurted out without even saying hello. I knew it was Jean because she was always angry with Bert, and even though she was

a good friend, I had "I'm-angry-at-Bert-fatigue." I finally cut her off between the part about his weight and the part about how the lawn needed mowing. "Look, Jean, here's the deal: either forgive him or divorce him, but never mention his name to me again." There was dead silence as the words I'd practiced over and over in my head were finally hanging in the air for all to hear. "I gotta go," I awkwardly mumbled, and then added, "I'm not trying to hurt you, but all this talk in five years has done nothing but use up our lives, and we both deserve more." My heart was pounding. Even if Jean never changed, I knew it was time for me to take back my life.

If you're reading this book, you're unusual. Unusual because many people who are disappointed with any part of their lives simply settle for that disappointment. Many people who are frustrated or frightened or in pain don't reach out to discover the source of that pain and are not willing to change. Many people don't do anything to remove whatever is blocking their lives. They don't believe they have power to change themselves, their circumstances or the outcome of their lives. Or the discomfort is just bad enough to make them realize they're unhappy—and sit around complaining for years—but not painful enough to really make them take any action.

There are so many reasons why people miss out on happy, productive, caring lives. Often these reasons stem from all the negative 'junk' ideas they were fed when they were younger. Stop and think. How did you feel about yourself at two years old? You probably thought you were the wisest, funniest, cleverest, cutest kid around. So what changed you? The opinions of others. Isn't it time we get our own opinions back?

Change Exercise 1

Watch a small child in action at the grocery store and notice how she or he operates:

How do children ask for things?

_____

What do they do if someone tells them *no*?

_____

How open are they to strangers who smile?

_____

Most children expect people will like them. They ask for something again and again. "No" only makes them more determined to get a "yes." They expect to get what they want. What happened to us? What most people do as they grow up is accept other people's opinion of their abilities, the world in general and their lives in particular. If someone says we can't play the piano, aren't good at art, can't sing or do math, we tend to believe them. Especially if we're small and they're big. We figure they must know better. We then try to numb our pain or frustration or anger at not being good enough. What we don't do is stop the outside messages or replace them with positive ones.

To deal with their disappointment, people may overeat, drink, deny it, do drugs, cheat, lie, stay out, stay in, do for others, do for themselves, forget it, dwell on it, go to class, read books or do anything in the world to try and get past their humiliation and pain.

Numbing ourselves is a great way to avoid the pain of anger or hurt, but the bad news is the pain of disappointment keeps coming back to haunt us unless we fix the root problem permanently. The constant noise in our head, the little voices that hit us just when we think we have things figured out, are the *Monster Lies* living inside our psyche, just itching to get out—but we're getting ahead of ourselves here.

So much of what has been limiting you—or downright stopping you—has to do with the beliefs that are floating around in your head like unchangeable truths. When, in reality, they're Lies (untruths) that have been fed to you by lots of often well-meaning, but misguided, people. When we buy these tenets as the "gospel," these comments sit and incubate. They become so real that we can't tell reality from fiction. Eventually we get so discouraged that we're sure there is absolutely nothing we can do.

Change Exercise 2

Think of three truths you were told as a child that are not true anymore: Example: All things come to those who wait. Pretty is as pretty does. Women are more suited for gentle professions like teaching or nursing. Good girls never raise their voices, etc.

1. _____

2. _____

3. _____

The real truth is that you've probably been carrying around these insidious Monster beliefs since childhood—or at least since adolescence. Getting kind of heavy, aren't they? They aren't real at all. They can be changed! You see, maybe the reason you don't have what you want isn't about your worthiness or ability or intelligence or common sense. Maybe it's about bad information you received somewhere along the way. That bad information has taught you to think in certain ways or to react to things in ways that get you stuck, not aware of all the options available for you.

Change Exercise 3

Now take a second and think of bad information you've been given by really well-meaning people. Examples: Work hard and keep quiet, someone will notice how smart you are. Look like you always have the answer and your boss will respect you. Act as if you don't care, men always love that.

1. _____

2. _____

3. _____

The problem is, most sources of information are only from educated guesses. Bad information is handed out as freely as good. Most times we've found bad choices aren't the result of being stupid. We make bad choices because we have bad information, poor data and limited know-how.

In addition, some very unpleasant things may have happened to you: someone you trusted and loved betrayed you; you got divorced; your parents got divorced; you couldn't afford to go to college; you were in an accident; you were abused; got very ill; were robbed; a loved one died; you got hooked up with drugs; or you lived a model existence and you still felt numb, empty and frustrated. Handling life's sorrows isn't easy, and it's worse with bad advice. Whatever has happened in your past, be it sad, regrettable—perhaps even tragic—you can overcome the past if you remember four things:

1. **No one is exempt from painful or frustrating experiences.** It's the cost of admission in this life. Even people who look happy have sadness.

2. **No one deserves to suffer. You can learn and reconstruct or you can dwell and self-destruct.** You don't have to suffer even if you think you deserve to because you brought it all on yourself. Here, however, you need to ask yourself what beliefs/Lies have convinced you that you don't deserve to have what you want.

3. **Pain is not a competition; it's a feeling.** No one has the right to judge whether or not your problem is worthy of pain or frustration. If you have pain, you have pain. You don't have to prove it's worthy enough for attention.

4. **What you do next about your problem, your pain, frustration, anger, unhappiness, will make the difference between having what you want in life versus continuing to suffer.** You have a choice. You can dig deep and find the root of your sadness, fear and disappointment. You can act in a way that helps you grow. Or you can try to bury the problem further with alcohol, self-created problems, drugs or work.

You can't control everything that happens in your life. What you can control is how you let it influence your future and how you problem-solve to reach the solutions you need.

Stop and think a second. What separates you from the star tennis player, the president of the student body, the CEO of your company, the mayor of your town or your incredibly happy friend? Not their money (sorry, but that's a lame argument, we both know too many very unhappy wealthy people), not their looks or talent or intellect. *It's their beliefs.*

Remember, everything you know about yourself is based on a belief you're holding. If you think you can be successful, happy, win the election, have great grades, maybe you can. If someone, or several someones, convinces you otherwise—and you accept that as truth—then you start to believe that you can't.

So in very simplistic terms, if we can control the *Monster Lies*—and they're very real, living creatures just waiting to sabotage us every chance they can—then there are truly no real limits as to what we can accomplish, do, have, feel and enjoy.

One reason we become overwhelmed with our problems is that we often think they're our fault. We believe there must be something wrong with us if we keep ending up making the same mistakes, or if we can't seem to get unstuck.

Sally

"Well, if you have an abusive boss," the wanna-be guru in the break room declared with a vacuous look in her eyes, "the universe must know you need this person to create a healing in your life, or take care of unfinished business from a past life." She assumed her pithy message was a gift. It cer-

tainly was not. "Life isn't hard enough sometimes," I pondered, "now I'm supposed to accept that I attract all these lunatics like some invisible caramel karma sauce all over my skin."

"Is it possible," I suggested, "that my boss is a raving alcoholic, and I'm the first person healthy enough not to put up with her very bad behavior?"

What is up with this "acceptance theory of life?" The one that says "everything" in your path is supposed to be there. Now we'll grant you that everything in our path, is in our path. Like walking on a rock jetty covered with seagull poop. It may be in our path, but we have no use for it, and we're stepping around it or letting the waves wash it away.

Some things are lessons, others are distractions. Shun the distractions!

We're not going to embrace it just because it's there. We're not going to punish ourselves with the thought we're drawing bad things toward us because we're not perfect yet. There's just a lot of negativity in the world, and it's hard not to step into it every now and then. Don't dwell on it, don't blame yourself, just sidestep it and move on. You don't go forward in life by reliving the past, but by making better decisions for the future.

Where did all the *Monster Lies* come from? Do you know what you did to bring them on? Well, maybe you were a considerate, polite child who listened to parents/teachers/aunts or an older sibling who warned you about the world. The message stuck. Maybe you doubted your own great intellect and talent because of some unthinking professor, minister, boyfriend, husband or Girl Scout leader. The point is, all you did to collect these *Monster Lies* is act as a magnet for others' fears, paranoia, envy and caring. You were a child soaking up whatever was out there as information. The result has limited your abilities to move past all this junk, and to have what you want and need.

Change Exercise 4

Just to show you how pervasive these Lies are, list seven statements you've heard since childhood, statements that can often seem deceptively like common knowledge. Examples: Bad news comes in threes. Talk about your good fortune and it will disappear . . . get the idea?

1._____

2._____

3._____

4._____

5._____

6._____

7._____

Again, the good news is by becoming aware of the *Monster Lies* and understanding how to delete them from your consciousness—or at least put them in retirement—you can maneuver past anything that stands in your way, whether it be financial, personal, physical or emotional. You will find you have very few real limitations when you vacuum out the past beliefs lodged in your head like so much junk mail.

The past tells us what *did* happen, but it cannot tell us

what *might* happen. Past thinking results in a lot of energy about facts and details that we already know. What if the best use of our time is to stop analyzing what happened in the past (that keeps repeating itself) and, instead, take two big steps:

REVEAL: Ask, "What am I afraid of or believe will happen to me if I change?" What is stopping you?

ACT: Ask, "What will I do now? What are all of the options?"

So often we've been given bad directions, sometimes by well-meaning people, but these directions stop us from getting where we want to be. Imagine you're in a tourist information center in Florida looking for a map of Orlando, but you accidentally picked up a map of Miami instead. If you don't notice it's the wrong map you could drive around lost for hours. You know where you want to be, but using the faulty information you were given, you aren't going to find your way there. Often that's what happens to us. We buy into the "directions" we get—from school, parents, television, newspapers—and it not only stops us from moving in the right direction, it practically paralyzes us from moving at all.

Now here's the *really big* question: Do you want to stop running in circles and get to where you want to be? Do you want a better map, better information and new ways to think? Do you want to finally quit repeating old behavior that isn't getting you where you want—or stops you from living and having what you really want out of life?

Change Exercise 5

Take five minutes to write out your secret vision. Even if you've done this before, answer these simple questions, keeping in mind that our lives always reflect our beliefs about what we can and can't do or have:

How much money would you like in the bank by next year?

_____

Who would you like to restore a relationship with? Who would you like to meet?

_____

What kind of car would you like to drive?

_____

Where would you like to live?

_____

Where would you like to travel to within the next ten years?

_____

What kind of love do you want in your life?

_____

The first step to controlling your destiny is to be very clear about what you would like to have changed. The alternative is things will stay pretty much the same. You can beat yourself up, continue to blame yourself, your financial situation, your friends, bosses, teachers, or any particular situation you're currently using as an excuse not to get on with your life.

You might blame your parents, cultural heritage, ex-spouse, gender, society, or bad karma, but it probably won't get you anywhere. You'll still stay exactly where you are. By the way, you may even have a right to blame them, but you will never get what you really want. Why? Primarily because your future will follow where you put your energy. If you put your energy into the past and relive all the hurts each day, then your future will look a lot like the past. If you put your energy and resources into your vision, giving up blame, your future will start looking like your vision. Pretty neat, huh?

So, are you ready to give up your pain, anger or frustration? Ready to stop being the victim and take total responsibility for everything that's going on in your life? Ready to experience real joy and peace in your life?

Of course, that means you need a more accurate map. With that map you can discover an easy way to get better information for your journey, a formula that actually helps you learn how to think smarter and more quickly and stop repeating the cycle. In this book we will offer a formula to finally deal with the *Monster Lies* that have plagued you and stopped you from being the person you know you can be. Of course, the best time to begin the journey is right this very minute. So, let's begin.

Change to What? What Do You Want?

Boom, ba-ba-boom. There was a rumbling thud in the playroom. The anxious new parents slowly peeked around the corner. There was a fifty-fifty chance their sixteen-month-old baby boy was fine. Often, he would fall over, pick himself up and go about his business. However, if he saw an anxious look in his father's eyes or he heard his mother scream, he would suspect there was something very wrong and start crying, even if he wasn't hurt.

Sometimes we expect that a certain chain of events should

be distressing, and we react out of fear before the actual impact. Physical pain comes from nerve messages to protect the body. Sometimes physical pain comes from fear or depression or anger. Most physical pain is the body's way of announcing there is a problem, like a burglar alarm.

Emotional pain, however, is more often the result of our thinking and our perspective than of bodily harm. It's caused by a gap between what we expected, planned and hoped for, and what we really got—which can be a downer.

Jennifer

I actually grew up in an era when the general consensus of many naive young women was that you didn't need to learn skills like cooking, because if you grew up and married well, you could afford to have someone else do the cooking for you. In this case, there wasn't just a gap between expectations and reality, there was a canyon that dwarfed that rather large one out in Arizona.

The further apart our lofty expectations are from our current disappointing experiences, the greater the pain. Often, the greater the guilt or frustration, the more we blame ourselves for not having what we expected to have by now.

You don't have to be a certain age to be frustrated with your expectations. You can be eighteen and starting college, but you don't have a full scholarship as you thought you probably would, considering your high grades and keen intellect. If that's not bad enough, what about all your relatives who are asking innocently why you don't have that scholarship?

Very often it can be something as simple as a forgotten birthday. We can be painfully disappointed if we assume our best friend will remember our birthday with a gift, card, lunch or dinner. If no one remembers, and we expect a celebration of sorts, there's a lot of room for disappointment.

Change Exercise 6

Imagine a clothesline with two clothespins (shown with a V) clipped on it, one at each end. One end is what you want; the other is what you ended up with.

What you've always wanted.   What you got instead.

V ◄━━━━━━━━► X ◄━━━━━━━━► V

Now as you move these two clothespins together, the gap (X) gets smaller and the distance between what you wanted and what you got gets smaller. For instance, you wanted chocolate chip ice cream, but you got chocolate almond ice cream instead. It's not what you wanted, but it's definitely closer than spinach *soufflé*.

The space between clothespins is not that great, so your disappointment will be limited to a quick pout. If the pins on the line are too far apart, it's like asking for chocolate ice cream and being told there are only cold sausages available. Between ice cream and sausages there's a really big difference. The pain is increased if you believe that you have no power to change your clothespins/reality. We all suffer if we feel we just have to "take it," "stuff it" or "accept it." We feel life has cheated us.

Jennifer

This gap between expectations and reality is one of the

35

SALLY FRANZ & JENNIFER WEBB

*main reasons for depression—the reason I wanted to sink
into a very deep hole and hibernate for about ten years while
my marriage was slowly decaying. I looked around and mis-
takenly thought I had no options, no power to change my reality. I can't think of anything more frightening and—in
retrospect—anything that was further from the truth.*

Lowering your expectations is not the answer. Many people have addressed the issue of emotional pain by suggesting
that if you lower your expectations to look more like your reality, you will experience less emotional pain. The idea here is
that if pain is caused by a huge gap between what you expected and what actually happens, expect less. Does expecting
less really lessen life's pain overall? Say you'll settle for dating
anyone who's halfway intelligent and reasonably attractive, so
you aren't disappointed with the blind date even though he's
light years away from what you were wishing for. Now what
if you marry Mr. Wrong? Forever until "death do us part" is a
long time.

But instead of lowering your expectations, what if you increased your reality? What if you actually started behaving in
ways that allowed you to get more of what makes you happy
every single day? What if you brought the two ends—the one
of reality and the other of expectations—together by moving
the reality pin closer to the expectation side: that is, by increasing what you really experience and have? What if, instead
of settling and making do, you created more of what you
wanted? You can, if you're willing to change some key beliefs.

These beliefs control how we expect reality to show up.
You see, we have some very specific pictures in our mind of
how our happiness should be fulfilled. These are taught to us
by our culture. When we learn to focus on our needs and let

go of the form or symbols of success, miraculous things begin to happen. Let's say you want to own a $150,000 sailboat because you love to sail. The problem is, you can only afford a $150 sailboat. There's some pain between your wishes and what is possible. There'll continue to be a large gap as long as you believe you have to own that sailboat in order to enjoy the sun and the water.

If what you love to do is sail large boats, there may a number of ways: you could crew, host weekend sail parties, cater aboard large vessels, etc. The key is to identify what you really like . . . sailing certain boats, sunshine, or perhaps telling people you own a big boat. If you really want to own that boat, then you may have to sacrifice other things and realign your priorities. You may have to work three jobs for ten years or take out a huge loan.

What do you really want?

Good question! Often, how we equate success is based on what we learned as children. We know this is true because country to country, town to town, class to class and family to family, there are strong cultural messages of what success is; what beauty is; who is in and who is out; who counts and who doesn't. We're taught that happiness is available when certain conditions occur or are met.

How else can you explain wealthy, talented, beautiful people—the American version of the right set of conditions to be happy—who are in psychological hell? Think of all of the big stars: John Belushi, Elvis, Janis Joplin, Jimmy Hendrix, Jim Morrison, Kurt Cobain, who couldn't cope with their lives. Then look at many people who are financially impoverished— the American definition of an absence of the correct conditions for happiness—who sing and laugh and have deep, enduring friendships.

The key to having all that you need and want to make you happy lies in understanding what really makes you happy versus what you've been trained to think *should* make you happy. Then get out the tools to have what you want. Those tools include understanding the cultural beliefs and Lies that keep you from happiness, and rethinking how you can use your resources to achieve your dreams.

You don't have what you want because you've believed these Lies. You've been taken in by very strong culturalization. We all believe a few strange ideas, not as if they're something we choose to believe, but as if they're the most sacred truths. Most of what we believe as "the Truth"—the right way to make a bed, the right way to park a car—we just assume everyone else also accepts as "the Truth." But that often is not the case.

Let's try a little experiment. Let's say all your family is gone, you're alone on your birthday, and celebrations are very important to you. You're afraid your friends at work will forget your birthday (an example of a painful disappointment).

You could have high hopes and likely be disappointed.

You could lower your expectations and not be disappointed—and also not get what you want.

Or you could try any of the following:

☞ What if this year for your birthday you bought a cake and streamers and arrived at the office . . . even sent a card around to be signed?

☞ Or you took yourself to a restaurant, or invited people over for a non-surprise party?

☞ Don't have any friends available right now? What if you went to a nursing home or hospital wing and threw yourself a party with a captive audience? You could make party hats out of newspaper funnies and crayons. You could make puppets out of paper bags. You could add everyone's name to the cake who had your same birthday month

Jennifer

I was walking down a street in New York when a quiet man handed me a slip of paper, looked into my eyes, said "Thank you," and kept walking. Assuming it was a solicitation for money I glanced at the paper, and it said simply, "I need a friend." It was signed, Bendu, *with a post office box number. Now my belief is that Bendu didn't know you could acquire friends from many different sources, and being in a strange city, in a strange country, he thought this approach might work. I wrote Bendu, suggesting he do a variety of things such as attend local churches, offer his time as a volunteer in certain organizations such as the ASPCA or the local Humane Society, or if possible he could adopt a pet.*

Do you have a belief that birthday parties only count if someone else throws them?

Do you have a belief that parties only count if you know the guests . . . that strangers won't do?

Do you have a belief that hanging out with sick or old people is not cool and doesn't represent your level of worth?

Come on now, be honest. Would you feel like a loser if you had to plan your own birthday celebration and spend it with

39

SALLY FRANZ & JENNIFER WEBB

people society might deem unacceptable? You know, the people you usually pity, not party with? What if you could throw a party and invite ten of your favorite celebrities? Ah, so maybe you would throw a party for yourself if cool people would come. Or maybe no matter who was there for you, someone else would have to plan it for it to "really" count. This experiment is your first lesson in finding out what the Lies are that control you and keep you from having a good time on your birthday. Negative beliefs steal happiness more than other people do.

Sally

"Who's going to take care of me?" I asked my therapist. The reply was simple: "You are."

How can I do special things for myself? I wondered. I can't throw myself a surprise party (unless I get hit on the head and have amnesia). I didn't think a birthday counted unless someone who loved me made the arrangements. I was brought up that way. Most of my childhood storybooks told of people or animal friends preparing celebrations for each other. There would be gooey vanilla icing dripping over a dark chocolate cake, and candy in cups. Anyway, many people told me it was poor form to throw one's own party. However, when I was forty, I was divorced, all alone, and knew that if I didn't create a new way to find happiness on my birthday I would be miserably alone. That was when I started throwing huge celebrations for myself. I also started taking myself on outrageous birthday trips during my birthday month . . . trips around the world. Clients paid for most of those trips. I figured out how to have the time of my life, and it didn't cost me more than the refreshments at the party.

I will admit that for the first few years I had a nagging voice (our Monster Lies *again) trying to convince me it didn't really count. But I'm proud to tell you I all but silenced that silly little voice. The result is, I love my birthday in whatever way I chose to celebrate.*

You can get anything you want in life if you begin concentrating on the innermost need, and let go of "how" it has to show up. Tear away the wrapping and get to the contents. Don't let local conditioning (Lies) keep you from happiness. Are you surrounded by Lies that keep you from being happy? These are some we've heard:

- *"I can't afford to go to Europe."* It still counts even if it's not a first class trip.
- *"I can't finish my degree."* There's no time limit on how long it takes. Even one course a semester will eventually yield you a degree.
- *"Self-published books don't sell."* Anthony Robbins was self-published.
- *"Adoption isn't the same as having a real baby."* No, sometimes it's better.
- *"I can't afford to live near the ocean."* Could you afford to house-sit an oceanfront cottage for pay?
- *"I'll never pay off my $10,000 credit card bill."* Why not start sending them $10 a month or seek mediation to resolve the debt?
- *"I can never stop dating men who are bad for me."* Exercise your right to choose. Slow down, be selective and keep in mind your own self-worth.
- *"I can't stop drinking."* Many people are sober thanks to AA.

Change Exercise 7

How do you discover what Lies are tricking you out of your happiness? It's easy. Just use this *Monster Lies*-Buster Exercise. Which *Monster Lies* are honored guests in the home you grew up in? Examples: You have to pay your dues. You: aren't old enough; don't have enough experience; don't have the education; are killing your mother; never get it right.

1. _____

2. _____

3. _____

4. _____

5. _____

Decide what you want right now that you don't have in your life: more friends; a job you enjoy; a love relationship; to lose weight; to have more money; to live in a better place; etc. Now write that particular desire down on the top of a blank page. Next, beneath that desire, write 1-10 in a column. Then start writing down all the things you can think of that will stop you from having what you want.

Inside the excuse is where the Lie lives. The Lies are so slick—so smoothly ingrained into our existence—that most of the time we don't have an inkling they are Lies. Topping most lists are: money, time, education, connections, love, skin color, gender, class, ability, age and/or luck. First ask yourself this: Who told you these things could stop you from having what you want? Then ask yourself this powerful and scary question:

What if these are just excuses and Lies passed on from one generation to the next?

Even if you have evidence these reasons are valid, is it possible you haven't experienced all there is in the world? Is it possible you haven't met everyone in the world, asked all the people in the world, and heard all of the stories in the world, that could enable you to have what you want?

Most of us have little (or big, gruff) voices in our heads. Some people refer to all these different voices as "the committee" or "the tapes." The fact is, we all know the voice; some say it is the child within and others say it's the old person within. We're talking here about the negative inner voice that keeps you locked in fear, or makes you feel lousy about yourself. This voice is the one that tells you not to try something, reminds you of all the really stupid things you've done throughout your life or that it's not worth the bother because it never works when you try it anyhow.

By the way, did you ever think you might continue the pattern of failure just because you're used to it, because it's a habit? It's just as easy—if not easier—to succeed as it is to fail? To have something not work requires all kinds of circumstances that have to be just right in order to miss opportunities. Our subconscious minds have to work very hard to keep our pattern of failure intact.

If you want to know what you really believe, just watch what you do. If you want to know what these voices say, just ask your brain to pull up the files. It's easy. Ask yourself a defeating question like, "How could I be so stupid?" Your "computer" brain will oblige you by pulling all references to stupid, humiliating, embarrassing, etc. Statistically these insidious little voices talk to us at a rate of 600 to 800 words per minute. Scary how much negative, infiltrating junk can be pumped into our heads at that rate. Keep this in mind: We, ourselves, are the most influential person we'll speak to during the day.

These voices are not—*we repeat*—not *your friends!* They do not represent the truth. Instead they represent partial facts about the past and have nothing whatsoever to do with the future! They speak with the authority of a scribe. They absolutely paralyze us from being effective. We might go ahead with plans and dreams, but with a defeatist attitude already in place. So who are these voices anyway?

What are the Missing Tools for Change?

"I'm here for the MENSA meeting," says Scott Adams's *Dilbert* cartoon character. It's early morning, 5:00 a.m., and Dilbert is standing outside the door talking to a man in his pajamas. "It's at 5:00 *p.m.!*" the annoyed host announces. Many people who appear to be smart with facts, figures and systems can be real dummies when it comes to everyday logistics or solving life's problems. Knowing a lot is not the same thing as perceiving a lot. True intelligence is a combination of information balanced with wisdom, experience and understanding. So strive for wisdom beyond knowledge and you will accomplish your goals.

Jennifer

I have two friends, one with a photographic memory and an IQ that seems to break all barriers. I don't know how many languages he speaks, but a typical conversation with him might start with an observation on anthropology. He comments on a time when he and Margaret Mead spent some time together in a tiny village . . . in a country I never

heard of, philosophies and cultures I've never heard of. And
he's genuine; it's all true.

I have another friend, a great guy who came from a very
poor family, dropped out before high school *and through*
hard work and guts carved out a successful business for him-
self. He's fun, interesting and smart. I mention these two be-
cause they're friends, and several times the second guy, the
one without a high school education, has gone over to his
friend's home (Mr. High IQ) to help with all kinds of
things, from plugging in a VCR (Note: I didn't say pro-
gramming, just plugging in, because Mr. IQ couldn't figure
out why it didn't work) to a myriad of other little things. So
IQ isn't the end all and be all.

The best way to outsmart these *Monster Lies* is to use our
minds creatively. In the past, most authorities looked at IQ to
determine intelligence, or they joined MENSA, an organization whose membership is based on IQ, to prove they were
smarter than most other people were. Intelligence was meas-
ured by what people knew, not what they could create.

In the 70s there was a version of an IQ test that suggested standard tests were more about your cultural background
than your actual intellectual potential. All of the questions in
this version were based on living in a black family raised in a
low income area. The result, of course, was that poor inner city
blacks who scored low on the traditional IQ test scored extremely well on the inner city culture IQ test. Whites from the
suburbs, on the other hand, scored very low.

IQ is relative. Why? Because the people making up the
test can use content out of their base of knowledge and experience. They deem that body of knowledge "the Truth," and
that is what they test for. In fact, the IQ test was originally

used to determine grade level for children. The only thing standard question-and-answer tests can measure is how well you can memorize the answers about a certain body of information. That, of course, is only part of smart thinking.

Thinking smarter has to do with researching more alternatives, combining existing knowledge with new applications, and using the basic properties of the brain to create new ideas and solutions.

Understanding that there are many approaches to any given situation is a sign of intelligence. The more options you create with language and your thinking, the more possibilities you have for right answers.

Today, thinking smarter has to do with new skill sets. Smart thinking is about the skills to problem-solve, brainstorm, rethink a situation, redesign a system for getting work done, negotiate and engineer emotions and feelings to get the best result for everyone involved. We define smart people as:

Those who train themselves to make good choices, which gets them the desired results.

Those who take full responsibility for their actions, because they don't believe in being victims, and have learned creative skills to be in control of their choices.

Those who avoid creating problems that demand all their time and energy, resolve conflict peacefully and have *fun*. They accomplish good things, and they give back to their community.

Those who don't simply take *no* for an answer because they're willing for the answer to take many shapes.

The smartest people are those who can create new ideas. The slowest people keep trying to do something the same old way and expect things to change because they're trying so hard. Most people are terrified things might actually change, which would set up a whole new set of problems. The effort of truly resistant people—defined as those who depend on society, the evening news and the *Monster Lies* to know how to act—goes into looking good, not changing the circumstances. They also like to look as if they're trying harder than people who are really making a difference. Slow people like to look smart, but that is quite different from being smart.

Jennifer

"You're fired," her boss said. "Gather your things from your desk and go see Personnel."

A friend of mine owned a small ad agency outside of Chicago, and when it became too much of a hassle, she eventually closed it down and joined a large, well-known firm in the city. The competition was very stressful for her, and finally one of the young men she hired and mentored was promoted over her. That's when he lowered the boom and downsized her out of a job.

Devastated, her entire life devoted to advertising, she decided to get smart. She decided to change professions, taking stock of what she needed to know and what she needed to have peace of mind and be happy. She focused on a career in nursing, which she had always wanted to get involved in, but had gotten sidetracked. With no background in the field—and very intimidated by science and math—she went back to school to get what she needed for a degree in nursing. By the way, she was fifty-seven years old when she made this decision, and today has happily settled into her new career. Traditional thinking wouldn't have allowed her to see the possibilities of changing professions.

It would've been very easy for her to become bitter and

disillusioned or to keep trying to get work in an area where she was comfortable. By acknowledging her old career was a dead-end, she was able to jump-start her life, and find the security and gratification she needed by moving in a completely different direction.

We're never too old. It's never too late. We can find ways to get where we need to be. Ask Moses or Grandma Moses. But if we try to solve problems based only on old information, we could very easily end up stuck. We've found there are always people out there who have experienced much worse than we have. They've created new lives for themselves by not accepting things the way they are, but by searching out new approaches to go after and get what they want. They center themselves, calm down, pray and start knocking on every door, asking for help, information and advice. With that mentality, the sky really is the limit.

So exactly who are the smartest people?

On the job, many businesses heap praise and rewards on employees who clock the longest hours, which doesn't necessarily have anything to do with thinking or working smarter or more quickly. It's not always the student who stays up till the crack of dawn studying, or the person who rehearses his part in the play longer or keeps rewriting the report until daybreak. The best and brightest in any capacity focus on how to work smarter, not longer.

Smart thinking can solve questions quickly because smart thinkers can get to the root of the problem sooner. Smart thinkers know what questions to ask and then know exercises to brainstorm innovative answers.

Change Exercise 8

A lot of the smart thinking techniques come from lessons in motherhood. Let's say you have two apples and five kids. How would you divide the apples so that it was fair?

_____

_____

The left-brain/analytical thinker may try to decide what percentage of apple each child will get. The emotional/right-brain thinker might determine who should get the apples based on performance and reward.

The smart thinker starts at a different place. She might look at the event from the eyes of an outsider—say an anthropologist, or an alien, or a child. Then her questions change. What are apples? Who eats them? Why? Maybe apples aren't for eating? Why not use the apples for bobbing, or dry the apples and make puppet heads, or make apple sauce, or sell the apples and buy enough ice cream for everyone, or have a game of peeling them and use the peels in an art project?

The smart thinker starts by asking: What are we doing here? Why do we do it that way? Is there another way? What do we all want? Why not use the apples for a non-food purpose? Does everybody here like to eat apples? Accelerated thinking points out the necessity for looking at any issue from an entirely different perspective: adding, dividing, creating different uses or answers by reshaping the issue. The same thing is true in smart thinking. We've been buying the old picture/problem/belief/Lie for so long we aren't even aware there are loads of other approaches.

It's a little like riding in a convertible for the first time. Suddenly, you're looking at the same old buildings you've passed your whole life, but in a new light. Lo and behold, there are cupolas, spires, domes, unique windows, birds' nests, and all sorts of other things you never imagined before. Why? Because suddenly you aren't looking at the buildings in the same old way; you have a new perspective with the top down. Here's the best news of all: anyone can learn these great new change skills. Everyone can learn to have superior thinking with powerful results, wisdom and success. All of us can conquer our *Monster Lies* provided we can identify the Monster and form an action plan.

REVEALING *Monster Lies* and acting to combat their negative influence will take courage and new thinking. You'll have to choose to ACT in ways that go against the familiar, but ordinary people can get extraordinary RESULTS.

CHAPTER THREE
The Monster Lie Doomsday

The Truth Doomsday doesn't want you to know:
Hold onto your hope—it's your key to the future!

W e're going to REVEAL how this Monster destroys your dreams and ruins your future by taking your hope—often insidiously in small ways of which you're unaware. We'll show you how to ACT immediately to regain control of your destiny, live every day filled with hope and do any- and everything you want to get the RESULTS you deserve, beginning right now, today.

Meet the Monster Doomsday

Even though no one really knows what tomorrow may bring, Doomsday can fill you with such dread and hopelessness you'll never have a great day. It likes to show up and kick you when you're down. If you have a temporary setback, It Lies to you that the situation is permanent. Doomsday likes to shame anyone who is positive into being more "realistic," more like It.

Doomsday always has evidence to substantiate Its case. It has the news media, talk shows, movies and all-important surveys and research labs where a few hundred people are interviewed, and then umbrella statements are made as if they apply to everyone, everywhere.

Doomsday tells us that tomorrow will be a slice of yesterday, so of course, it's hard to get excited about the future. Constantly dwelling on the past doesn't help us create a better tomorrow. It's one thing to learn from the past—take the best, leave the rest. It's another thing to live there.

Doomsday's Voice

We all hear the voice of Doomsday everywhere we go. It's a monotone; a lifeless, apathetic whisper often trailing off in despair. It's in the culture; It's in the music—especially Country and Western music. Doomsday is in your head. Have you ever heard these words before?

It always turns out the same.
Why keep hitting your head against the wall?
No matter how hard you try, you fail.
You're a loser.
Broke again and at your age!
You'll never make anything of yourself.
You're a nobody; always have been, always will be.
This relationship is never going to change: you're stuck.

Doomsday Exercise 1

Okay, it's your turn. What does Doomsday say to you when you're down? Who do you know who uses Doomsday to hold you down? Remember it's often the little innocuous words that do the most damage.

<u>*Example*</u>
Doomsday says: *"You'll never amount to anything."*
Who's speaking: *My father*

Doomsday Says:_____

Who's speaking:_____

Doomsday Says:_____

Who's speaking:_____

Doomsday Says:_____

Who's speaking:_____

Doomsday Says:_____

Who's speaking:_____

Doomsday Says:_____

Who's speaking:_____

Doomsday Says:_____

Who's speaking:_____

Visualizing Doomsday

Now comes the fun part: attacking this Monster. We're going to make this most damaging *Monster Lie* look like a cartoon, to ridicule and humiliate this creature because It's no friend. The more ridiculous the better, because we'll be reminded not to listen to It or take It seriously.

This is how we picture Doomsday: Imagine a large purplish-brown raccoon with a human-like face, squinty eyes with dark circles beneath them (because of all its worry and gloom) and a long pointy nose. Arrogant and unconcerned with your pain, It wants you to stay defeated—a victim, a doormat, a failure. It's always insisting nothing ever changes and nothing ever gets better. It smells like rotting leaves and onions. Its fur is coarse and prickly. You know you don't want to be near It for very long.

How Does Doomsday Limit You?

It tells us we can't possibly change the direction of our life because it'd take too great an effort to really get results. It sounds so logical! *Beware!* The Lie is this—that only a huge miracle will save us. This "realistic" thinking tricks us into submission; often we give up without even trying. This belief makes us blind to the simple truth that the small changes and choices we make every day can create a world of difference.

The cumulative effect of these small choices can yield the miracles we need, but when we don't see any immediate changes happening, we often give up in despair, convinced that "all is lost." It doesn't occur to us that things are simply delayed. We give up waiting for our ship to come in, convinced it has already sunk with no survivors. In the business environment we hear this mentality every day:

> *"What's the use? It won't matter anyway."*
> *"Guaranteed the company won't go for it, so why bother?"*
> *"It'll just get shot down, so don't waste your time."*
> *"We already tried that. It doesn't work."*

This attitude, this belief system, is so insidious it's like an invisible plague. (It should be mandatory to get an inoculation against this pervasive thinking—have you had your all-is-hopeless-and-there's-nothing-to-live-for shot yet?) It stifles creativity and leads to despair, lethargy and depression, because if we think a situation is hopeless, then we've nothing left to fight for. Take away the ability to hope, and you've taken away one of the most valuable emotions and motivations we possess.

Often we decide something ought to be done, that it's time for a drastic change in some part of our lives. Then we try to undo twenty years of conditioning overnight, and we're extremely annoyed when we mess up. "Typical," we think. "Just like me. I never could pull it off." Neither could anyone else if faced with such a huge task.

Be patient with yourself. Understand that most great changes in life occur so softly, so subtly that you aren't aware they've taken place. If you focus on an idea, a project, an exercise routine, a new approach, just five minutes a day for two weeks, then you'll see the seeds take hold, grow and begin to bloom.

Think about it. Would you tackle an enormous project that seemed overwhelming and infinite all at once? Or would you prefer to deal with something in segments where you could actually envision reaching a small goal, a small plateau?

There's the old tale of the father who taught his son how to have the strength to lift a cow. It didn't begin with weight lifting or conditioning routines. It began with lifting a calf. The calf was tiny and easy to lift. Every day, twice a day, the son was required to lift the calf. Little by little the calf grew into a cow. Gradually, little by little, the son's strength grew accordingly.

SALLY FRANZ & JENNIFER WEBB

Facing the Monster Doomsday: Our Stories

Sally

"I know you, and no one will ever love you!" shouted my ex-husband.

"There aren't any nice men left for you," moaned my grandmother.

"You must be having a breakdown to leave such a nice man," my mother added.

"Divorce must be French for pain," I thought.

No matter where I turned, I was reminded of what a failure I was, and most likely would continue to be. The shock of starting over was hard enough, but my biggest enemy was myself. The voice inside my head said, "You're a complete and total idiot. You have failed God and your children and your church and your community, and you deserve to be miserable, and a long and torturous death wouldn't be a surprise." It was as if the Monster Lie Doomsday had a crystal ball, and the future was always bleak and cloudy.

Jennifer

Once I found myself in the position where I was given two weeks to vacate my house. My husband and I had just divorced, and I'd been evicted. It was so overwhelming, I can't begin to tell you. There was just no way—"no how"—that this could be done. I had two small children and very little help. It seemed as if I would surely crumble under the weight of the tasks at hand.

But I broke it down into little pieces. I began by finding a rental property in town and a friend with a pickup truck. Then I decided to move my children's toys and furniture, and what I just had to have for myself. I worked methodically, deciding what I could leave if I had to. Little by little we saw progress, and within two weeks, I was in a small house with the most important items.

Don't try to "forecast." Stay with today. Or if today is too painful or overwhelming, stay with the morning. If the thought of all morning is too long—and we've been in this place before—just make it through an hour at a time. That you can do. Then deal with just the afternoon. Don't even dwell on evening until 6:00 p.m. rolls around.

Sally

In the middle of the Vietnam War, at a time in the 60s with consumerism rising, Lady Bird Johnson had a dream: "What if we could spread wildflowers along our highways and stop littering?" As a forerunner to Earth Day, Lady Bird's beautification project was launched in 1968 with leaders from twenty or more youth organizations such as Girl Scouts, Future Farmers of America, 4-H and YWCA. I went to Washington as a YWCA teen leader, and remember vividly how impressed I was with Lady Bird. Instead of seeing all of us as just teenagers, unable to make much difference in the world, she shared her vision of a more beautiful planet, and sent us out to create change. Her impact on me was so great that, twenty years later, I was on the advisory board of UNEP (United Nation's Environmental Program) and am still active in environmental programs today.

SALLY FRANZ & JENNIFER WEBB

Doomsday Exercise 2

Now it's your turn. Think of a really big task that seems improbable or impossible for you to do. Go back to college, pay for your child's braces, landscape the yard, create a report, or plan that national conference. Now break it into tiny little steps and do one or two a day.

Task

_____

Step 1 _____

✓ Completed by _____

Step 2 _____

✓ Completed by _____

Step 3 _____

✓ Completed by _____

Step 4 _____

✓ Completed by _____

Step 5 _____

✓ Completed by _____

Step 6 _____

✓ Completed by _____

Step 7 _____

✓ Completed by _____

Step 8 _____

✓ Completed by _____

Warning: Doomsday wouldn't be so destructive if It weren't so hard to spot. People are tricked into thinking Its pessimism is actually realism. Even if you can quiet the voices in your head, Doomsday inhabits the bodies of others—almost like an evil alien from another galaxy—and boy, does it hurt when It talks to us through a trusted friend or colleague.

Doomsday shows up in families, in college dorms, on work teams at the office, in places of worship and in boardrooms. In fact, It shows up any place where someone is suggesting a change in the way things are done. People resist change because they're afraid they won't be able to control the future and because they're afraid it will be worse than the present. "Better the devil you know," goes the saying.

People are also resistant to new ideas and dreams because if those new ideas just happen to work, it may mean they've wasted a lot of precious time doing something the "wrong way." They have a lot invested in the way things are. It's quite common for you to hear the voice of Doomsday from people in every part of your life, and the refrain is always the same: "Forget it, don't try it, why waste your time since it will never work."

Think rubber band! People resist change in much the same way our body resists change. The state of equilibrium is known as homeostasis. If our body is suddenly five degrees hotter, it will do its best to snap back to the correct body temperature. If it's four degrees cooler, it'll again snap back to the correct body temperature, much like a thermostat. Homeostasis doesn't just affect how our body operates to keep us safe and healthy; it can also operate in a home, an office, and a country.

The body knows change can be uncomfortable, painful, exhausting, boring, and possibly many other things. Therefore, it'll fight you if you don't take control. You must will yourself to continue with the change because it is ultimately very good for you, even though it feels lousy and uncomfortable.

Jennifer

Many years ago, I was a photojournalist. While I never developed my own film, I was an accomplished photographer. Later, I took a course in developing film, built a small darkroom and had fun with it as a hobby. Now, several years went by, and I was interviewed for a job that required extensive developing skills. I needed the job, I knew I could learn, and so I said yes, I could certainly do what was required.

I can still remember my first day on the job. After I was introduced to all my new coworkers, my boss took me to the darkroom door, handed me several rolls of film and started to walk away. At that moment I broke into a cold sweat. I couldn't begin to remember the steps to develop film, so I quickly explained I felt I was a little rusty, didn't know their facilities, and would he walk me through it once. I took copious mental notes, stayed late that night trying to remember what I needed to know, and got along just fine.

Had I admitted the truth that, no, I'd never utilized this one particular method, I may not have gotten the job. I'm certainly not recommending being deceitful, I'm simply saying there are many, many ways to get a job done, but often we have the knee-jerk "No" reaction to a question that limits our possibilities. If you face that situation, just ask the person hiring you what they need and then tell them what you need to help them get the job done.

Most employers are delighted with someone who can admit mistakes and ask for help. If they expect you to be perfect the first try, it's probably just a matter of time before you'll have to leave that job. Good employers want to know: Can I count on you to do the job?

Sally

"Great, there's a sale on the stomach medicine I use when I feel nausea coming on. I'll take three bottles."

Every time I've made a major leap forward in my life by sheer will, I've gotten physically sick. In fact, if I'm going to attend a new class, buy a new car, move or submit an article to a new editor, I just go buy a bottle of antacid or diarrhea medicine. I take charge of my body. I do not coddle myself and say, "uh-oh, this change is too hard or rapid." I slug down the chalky pink sludge, and my stomach is back to normal. We fight change even when we're the ones who decide to do it. How much more resistance can you expect from others—who don't want you to change? A lot!

Get the idea? People will fight, argue, pontificate, explain and do anything to keep from having to deal with change— even though it's the best thing for them. So, if you're fighting change, know it's a natural process to attempt to stay in exactly the same place. Understanding and acknowledging this will allow you more patience and determination in moving forward. Change makes us feel vulnerable, but staying in an unfulfilling place can be more dangerous. Not using our gifts is a waste.

Doomsday thrives where people have been knocked for a loop through loss, tragedy or poor performance. We know there has to be change, but we're afraid of it. That's when Doomsday sneaks around and dampens spirits. Just when you're totally drained and zapped, when you need a lift, Doomsday sits on your feet like cement slipper socks. You need inspiration, and there It sits reciting every known reason why you're going to fail. What have you tried to change before and still have trouble with? Like the guy who says it's easy to quit smoking, he's done it hundreds of times. We all have areas we struggle with.

Jennifer

One of the characteristics of Doomsday is It saps your strength and courage, the why-bother-it-can't-be-changed-anyway mentality. When I met and spent some time with actress/singer Ann-Margaret after her performance at Radio City Music Hall, I was impressed with how much she genuinely loved meeting and talking with new people. She was definitely in her element, and she loved it. Had she listened to Doomsday, I wouldn't have been talking with her that evening, considering years earlier she was in a tragic backstage accident that required a lot of surgery before she could make public appearances. Overcoming great odds, she pushed forward to perform again. If you listen to the voice that says you can't do it/repair it/try it, you'll be doomed before you begin.

Doomsday Exercise 3

List three areas in which you're resisting change.

Example
Thing I want to change: *I want to learn the computer.*
Doomsday says: *"You're too old for high tech."*

Thing I want to change:_____

Doomsday says:_____

Thing I want to change:_____

Doomsday says:_____

Thing I want to change:_____

Doomsday says:_____

Do you hear yourself saying: *I'm not being fatalistic; I'm being sensible?* *After all,* you rationalize, *this is the way it is. There's nothing I can do about it. I'm being honest with myself. I'm being pragmatic, reasonable. I see it as it really is.*

Stop! These sound so logical, who could even argue? But beware! You must resist giving in to these thoughts, because this is the food Doomsday thrives on. Don't nourish hopelessness. You need to go out and find proof that your dreams are possible. Because they *are* possible.

Imagine your dreams and goals represented in a beautiful, rolling lawn in front of the palace of your desires and beliefs. Now out there on the lawn, Doomsday has planted a nasty, negative weed. If left alone, the weed begins to choke out every pleasant blade of green grass in sight, every hope and dream. We don't even notice it at first.

Then, when we do notice, we start rationalizing. Okay, it's annoying, and it's not as pretty as the lawn, but it *is* green and—from a distance—it all blends in. "I'm too tired to go pulling out every negative thought by the roots. I'd have to get on my hands and knees and dig deep and then walk it over to the dumpster. I'll let it grow." (I won't make a call or ask for a job interview.)

Eventually the lovely lawn that was healthy and lush is a nasty pile of brown weeds that grow up around your dreams and your self-esteem and suffocate them. You've spotted Doomsday if you believe defeat is permanent, and that you're too powerless to uproot it. If you believe "nobody understands how I feel" or "this problem is even too big for God," you've probably been bitten by Doomsday and don't even know it.

Doomsday lives inside the words "What's the use?" Remember, if you nurture the weeds, they will grow. If you root them out and focus on the positive, even when it seems the most difficult thing you've ever done, then the green grass—the positive—will begin to grow.

"Yes, I can and yes, I will, so help me God!"

The problem is you haven't done enough research. You need to find out how other people have kick-started their dreams from the same place as where you are. One of the biggest drawbacks is we often haven't actually seen someone do it—break free of Doomsday and move forward, so we don't believe it can happen. That's why families repeat the cycle of poverty. They haven't seen anyone break free, and they're following the only available role models they have.

It's been proven that the most successful people are those who simply keep on. They take *no* out of their vocabulary.

Those who will not give up, but do one small thing—however small that thing happens to be—every single day, are the ones who succeed. For example, Oprah Winfrey didn't become a world-famous celebrity overnight. First she overcame a destructive childhood, then she got involved with TV. After creating the *Oprah* television show, she went on to star in the movie, *The Color Purple* and has since starred in and produced several more movies. She launched the renowned magazine, *O*. The key to her success? Keep on keeping on, and to remain gracious and caring to her public.

Just recently Oprah stopped into a dress shop in southern California. When the salesperson (a good friend of Sally's) saw who it was, she immediately gave Oprah a copy of her recently released self-help book, declaring that Oprah was a major inspiration in her own life. Oprah was encouraging and positive, just what this young writer needed to continue her work.

Calvin Coolidge said, "Nothing in the world takes the place of persistence. Talent will not. Nothing is more common than unsuccessful men with talent. Genius will not. Unrewarded genius is almost a proverb. Education will not. The world is filled with educated derelicts. Persistence and determination alone are omnipotent." Keep on despite what you're telling yourself, despite what evidence you see to the contrary, despite what friends tell you. The results will absolutely astound you!

Don't discount your every effort. We're so conditioned to look for the big picture, the big lottery win, that when we make an inroad, the first thing we do is discount it. "Oh, sure I took a course, but I still don't have a better job . . . see, nothing works."

Have you ever tried filling up a big jug of water? At first you think there is a hole in the bottom because it doesn't look like the water level is changing. Then—*whoosh*—it gets up to the narrow neck and in a flash pours over the top. We want the jug to overflow the minute we start filling it, yet it doesn't work that way. It won't fill at all if we spend our time upset that it takes so long and never even put it under the faucet.

Often, if we've taken little steps, we get discouraged and just stop, or take them back, feeling foolish that we even tried. Maybe you started college twenty years ago and are saying, "No way can I go back and finish. It's too late for me." Maybe you were learning to type, or ski, or master a new software program on the computer. You can still do whatever you want to do.

Remember the game "Mother May I?" You can only move if you remember to ask, "Mother, may I take three steps forward?" The real question isn't "Mother, may I?" But, "Self, may I go ahead with my life now?" The answer is . . . "Yes, you may." There's no one else to ask but yourself, because no one else can do it but you. No one else counts, no one else has the authority to give you permission, not even your mother.

Doomsday Exercise 4

Right now give yourself permission to be great. Give yourself permission to finish something big, or to make a big change in your life.

I give myself permission to:

_____

I give myself permission to:

_____

I give myself permission to:

_____

I give myself permission to:

_____

Now give yourself permission for this to take as long as it takes with baby steps.

I give myself permission to take as long as necessary to:

_____

I give myself permission to take as long as necessary to

_____

I give myself permission to take as long as necessary to

_____

I give myself permission to take as long as necessary to:

_____

Maybe we've all been eating instant food too long. Take it out, nuke it—*wham!* Potatoes *au gratin* in three minutes; tasting more like potatoes *au* rotten. When we don't get instant results, instant gratification or an immediate payoff for our investment, we freak out. We decide "it's" not going to work after all. Whatever the "it" is, we whine, complain and stop our forward movement. And the clock keeps right on ticking. We think little steps take too long, so we opt for the chance we'll win the lottery, or something major will suddenly come into our lives and rescue us. We just keep on waiting.

The best way to see if Doomsday has been around the home or office is to see how people are feeling about the future. Ask people:

"Where do you want to be in five years?"

"What three things do you want that would make your work easier?"

Jennifer

In my seminars I often ask participants to create the ideal work day: how would their commute be, where would their office windows face, what exciting work would they be doing? After they complete the exercise I ask them what would have to happen to have that in their lives right now, and what steps, beginning today, can they do to start creating that reality.

It doesn't happen in big chunks. It doesn't usually happen with luck or a serendipitous occurrence. It happens by taking the first step, by starting to move. Once you're in action, your life will start a gentle shift toward your dreams. Then one day you look around, and you've arrived. But while the effort is steady, it's not overnight.

Sally

"This is the worst gift I've ever gotten!" I cried.

I remember when Doomsday was sitting on my back, sapping all my energy. I was newly married, and we were really broke all the time. At the end of the month we had enough money left over so one of us could go to a movie, but you'd have to walk because there was no gas money.

That Christmas my mother sent me a gift. I still remember tearing off the wrapping, taking one look at the gift and bursting into tears. It was a suitcase, and it felt like a cruel joke to me at the time. I was so broke I "just knew" that I'd never be able to use that suitcase. That I'd never, ever have the money to travel anywhere again. That was in 1973.

I have long since worn out that suitcase. In the last five years I've traveled to Africa, Uzbekistan, Scandinavia, Europe, China, Manila, Banff, to Antigua on a cruise to see the total eclipse of the sun, to the Caribbean, Cancún, Catalina, Canada and to Costa Rica for a month of Spanish lessons. And to think, I couldn't even imagine traveling just three hours away in 1973.

You simply don't know what's around the corner, but it's worth the steps it takes to get there.

Doomsday Exercise 5

The best way to deal with Doomsday is to practice shedding despair and putting on hope. Remember that Doomsday is all around you, so you'll have to practice this quite often.

Take your problem: a lemon car, not enough money for tuition, a tough decision, loneliness, a problem child or whatever is causing you the most stress and feelings of hopelessness and despair. Then make a magazine montage—tear pictures from a magazine and glue them to a piece of plain paper. Put pictures of all the things you want and need for your situation to improve. Getting your right brain/creative side in gear does wonders to build hope and teach your left brain/analytical side how to identify the solution when it's near. Then look at this image on a daily basis. Lift it up in prayer or meditation. Focus on the needed answers and source for answers as often as possible.

Doomsday Exercise 6

We're in such a habit of saying *no* to new ideas that it is an automatic, knee-jerk reaction. Say *yes* to any and every "crazy" idea you hear this week. Or at least say, "I'll give that some thought."

Doomsday Exercise 7

Write down something you want. (This is Project Management 101.)

——————————————————————————

——————————————————————————

Now break it into baby steps. Put dates on the completion of those steps, and tell at least one person your goal. Now work on three things on your list every day—even if it's the same three things—until you make them happen. Create a habit just like brushing your teeth or taking your vitamins. Find ways to reward yourself for making a promise to yourself—and keeping it.

Sometimes the way you move mountains with faith is to find a little faith every day to get up and continue shoveling, no matter how insurmountable the project seems.

Doomsday Exercise 8

Celebrate now!

You've got to celebrate all the little stuff all the time. So many of us wait until a project is complete to celebrate. Imagine if the folks who worked on the pyramids did that? "Oh, I know you worked fifty years in suffering on this business, but only your grandchildren will get to celebrate."

Doomsday doesn't want you celebrating, because It doesn't want you to recognize the power of the little steps. If you think only the goal counts, It can defeat you.

Get out the real plates, silverware, bake a pie, or put jam on a piece of toast and put a candle in the middle of it. Buy yourself a card or a car—but celebrate life every week! If you're single, call up a friend and brag about what you've accomplished. If you're married or have kids, have a special dessert to celebrate your accomplishment. People rarely refuse to celebrate other people's accomplishments if there's food involved!

Why do these games work? Because these "games" are a way to dislodge Doomsday from your environment and allow good things to happen. You have to take charge. Your attitude and your ability to change your beliefs is the best lever there is to get problems off your back.

Be aware that the first steps in the tunnel toward the light may be in total darkness, and sometimes you'll be all alone. In fact, you'll be walking in darkness and heavy shadows for a while. The light at the end of the tunnel isn't a switch that brightens the place all at once. It's a gradual awareness that the worst is over. This piece of knowledge is all you need to get going and keep going. It's enough to keep Doomsday at bay for a long time.

Doomsday Exercise 9

☞ Every time you get the message you can't have what you want, go find three people whose dreams have come true.

☞ Ask the librarian for biographies of people who have succeeded despite the odds.

☞ Study famous people. What did they have to overcome and how did their attitudes get them where they wanted to be?

☞ Find someone to talk with who's overcome some obstacle. How did that person find the strength to continue?

Granted we can't talk to all our heroines. Harriet Tubman—the slave credited for helping others escape bondage by fleeing to the North via the network of safe houses called the Underground Railroad—had every excuse not to become the amazing social reformer and feminist who transformed so many lives. "I grew up like a neglected weed—ignorant of liberty, having no experience of it," she said in an 1855 interview with educator and part-time journalist Benjamin Drew. However she chose not to rely on all the reasons why a slight, black woman growing up during a period of profound racial upheaval couldn't make a difference, or overcome serious obstacles to her success.

Jennifer

Recently I sat next to a young woman on a plane as we landed on a Friday evening in Reno, Nevada. It was the height of ski season, and I asked her if she was planning to go skiing. She told me she lived close by and had just been back visiting her relatives in Ohio. As I listened to her story, I became more and more impressed. She was putting herself through school and—like so many other students—had no financial support from anyone and no money. So she decided last summer that while working for a rafting company by day, she would camp out in a tent on their grounds all summer in order to save money for tuition. Was it difficult and uncomfortable and lonely, I wondered? Her response was: it was what she'd needed to do in order to go to school, and she decided to make it work. The great news is there are many, many people like her out there, willing to share their stories and their passions for overcoming whatever stands in their way in order to live their dreams.

One way you tame Doomsday is to discover what you really want in life and determine you're going to get started on having it. Learning how to visualize a great tomorrow takes guts, work and a clear picture of what would make you happy. But the rewards are worth the effort. Watch one fewer TV show; get the kids to pitch in with the dishes while you read; reduce your internet time by ten percent.

Dare to dream big and fight off Doomsday. After all, It doesn't really know what tomorrow will bring; It just acts that way to upset you. You'll never get what you want if you don't dare to think big and dream what you really want to have in your life. Then don't discount that dream just because Doomsday—or even your own negative voice—jumps in to remind you it's not practical, realistic, feasible, do-able, logical. You'll never know until you try.

Doomsday Exercise 10

Every time you think about a negative problem, try to re-paint it in bright, bold colors. If you hate your boss, visualize her in a pink polka-dot vest and bright green shoes. If that's the way she dresses, then visualize her in silver leather motorcycle riding garb. This will give you some freedom to unhook from the sadness and pain of feeling trapped. If you can approach these situations creatively, then you can release your brain to problem-solve good solutions. It makes what you fear less powerful.

It also helps you to separate the problem from the person. You can't address the problem logically if you spend all your energy defending yourself from the person. Try to see the person as one thing and the problems and attitude he or she presents as something else.

Remember, no one owns your thoughts. You have the right to imagine and go beyond your wildest dreams. Don't waste energy giving others power to ruin your dreams.

Reminders

Ask yourself this:

- *What's the worst thing that could happen? And then what will happen after that?*

- *With what you've got right now, what kind of life could you build?*

- *Who could help you if the bottom drops out?*

- *Who would you help?*

- *Can you help each other? Why or why not?*

- *What will you lose if you try to get help?*

- *What is horrible right now, and how can you immediately begin to create change?*

☞ *What will happen if you do nothing?*

☞ *Do you want the rest of your life to be just as it is today?*

How do you outsmart Doomsday?

You start to look at the problem differently. Our questions and exercises are designed to build your thinking power and help you realize your potential while shortening your learning curve by miles. You slow down your assumptions by asking questions and re-examining where you got your beliefs. All of your experiences are little files. Some of them may not be accurate.

Your Action Plan

What are you afraid to hope for in the future, and why? What do you dare not hope for? List here:

_____

_____

List three steps to research how others achieved a similar dream (go to the library; cold-call someone successful; read biographies; ask for help):

1._____

2._____

3._____

Now do one of these three things immediately (within the next hour if possible), and preferably all three before you

---

read the next chapter.

Try these quick exercises to break Doomsday bad habits:

✓ Instead of saying *no* to a new and crazy idea; ask "Why not?"

✓ Ask: "What could happen if I did it anyway?"

✓ Ask: "Who could help me make this happen?"

✓ Ask: "Who believes in me, and who would be glad if this did happen (and can they help now)?"

✓ Ask: "What will this cost financially, emotionally, time-wise?"

✓ Ask, "Can I cover any expenses through barter or trade?"

✓ Ask: "Who has done something like this before?"

✓ Ask: "Who will suffer if I don't do this?"

✓ Don't assume you know the answer; ask: "How can I be sure?"

Be right on this one, and silence Doomsday's ugly voice full of fear and hopelessness. It is not your friend, so don't entertain one moment of Its pessimism.

Next, list the one thing that—if you could change it—would have a major impact on your life. Immediately list all the reasons people will remind you this isn't realistic. On a separate piece of paper, list ten things you can do, one each day or one every other day, to start making this a reality.

The Change:

_____

1. _____

2. _____

3. _____

4. _____

5. _____

6. _____

7. _____

8. _____

9. _____

10. _____

Summary

We've REVEALED that all those voices you've heard—often in such subtle whispers you thought they were your own ideas—have been responsible for stopping you. Remember it's not your fault if you've been fed these Lies, but it is your responsibility to overcome them.

How? By ACTING immediately, today. Take one or two small steps, and while you're at it, try something to demonstrate instant results. For half an hour only, do not allow one negative thought, one Doomsday thought, one Lie into your consciousness. Every time you hear a negative idea say, "Not now." You'll be amazed how many times you'll have to say those words. You'll be amazed at the RESULT—how liberating it feels when you control that negative impulse. Success is not an accident; it's an awareness.

We're not saying to ignore real problems. We're saying you'll pretty much be worthless as an effective problem-solver and powerhouse if you're burnt-out with hopelessness, fear and discouragement. You have to give your brain downtime from the problems and harshness of this world. You have to think about goodness, beauty and what may be possible. It will do you no good when your ship comes in if you sleep in late, saying, "Ships never come to my harbor." Get up and go down to the harbor every day, expectantly scanning the horizon. Not every sail you see will be yours, but what if you stop looking and miss yours?

Life is what you make of it. When you're right in the middle of something difficult, it's impossible to imagine there's a way out or around your situation. The truth is, there's not just one way, but possibly ten or twenty. Many women before you have struggled with the same issues and found solutions. Pat yourself on the back for what you've already done, and remember there are so many more opportunities out there for you—many you haven't even begun to imagine.

CHAPTER FOUR
The Monster Lie Stressor

The truth Stressor doesn't want you to know:
No one drives you crazy—you drive yourself there!

W e're going to REVEAL how this Monster causes you constant discomfort and eats away at your peace of mind by pressing all the little buttons that stress you out. Because stress is self-inflicted, we'll show you new ways to ACT. The RESULT will be that you'll be able to handle and reduce stress as soon as you recognize you have a choice, and follow through.

Meet the Monster Stressor

If you've spent a lot of time in your life believing that other people have control over your life, there's good news and bad news. It's the same message: you're completely in control of your life. No one makes you do anything. You do what you do to avoid feeling like the bad guy, or because you believe others have power over you if you don't. Unless you're on a Mafia hit list—and the Witness Protection Program isn't interested in shielding you anymore—you're the cause of your own stress and you can do something about it. Most of us, however, give away our power, placing blame somewhere else. Ever hear someone—including yourself—say:

You drive me crazy.
You make me so mad.
You've ruined my life!

Stressor's Voice

Stressor's voice is a raspy, stuck CD reminding you constantly of the mounting pressures you have no control over. It sounds like this:

You'll never get this all done by 5:00 p.m.
It's starting to snow; you'll get stranded.
You'll never manage to read all the assignment on time;
you'll probably fail.
You should have more done by this time.
You can't do this report on the old machine.
Everybody else is really dressed up; you look a mess.
What if something horrible happens?
All this traffic; you'll be late and you'll be fired.
Now that you've missed the flight, you'll miss the big meet-
ing, and your life will be ruined.

Stressor Exercise 1

Okay, now it's your turn. What does Stressor say to you?

1. _____

2. _____

3. _____

4. _____

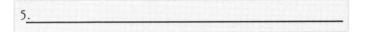

5.

Visualizing Stressor

Think of a big, jowly creature with frizzy orange hair and a grumpy, sagging mouth. Its hands are waving, Its eyes are darting back and forth frantically beneath furrowed eyebrows. It wants you to know there are big problems in this world, and you're surrounded by most of them.

Stressor wants you to believe you have no choice. If you buy Its propaganda, you probably don't. After all, bosses, teachers, spouses, children, and in fact, all of society have told you how you should behave and what you should believe. Trying to make everyone happy is a full-time job accomplished by no one. You are accountable to yourself.

The most important thing Stressor wants you to ignore is the fact that you have choices all the time. Operating from the knowledge that you have choices goes a long way toward reducing your level of stress.

Stress is what happens when reality shows up and ruins your plans. Stressor wants you to ignore reality and cling harder to your plans, which will enable you to act very stupidly. You'll drive too fast, fly in bad weather, raise your blood pressure, binge, cry, or yell at innocent people. We know! We have been snowed in at airports and listened to stressed-out passengers screaming at gate attendants to get those planes in the air! It doesn't matter if air traffic control says they're grounded! We create our stress by what we continually tell ourselves—or avoid stress by understanding the choices we have.

We can become unglued or we can reassess the options. In Game Show language . . . if you don't like what's behind Curtain Number One, and you don't know what's behind

Curtain Number Three, then pick Number Two! Don't stew all day about the other two choices.

How Does Stressor Limit You?

So often it's because we believe we're the exception to the rule. Sure, others may have choices, but we feel our problems are too overwhelming, so unique there just are no answers. We feel beaten down and powerless.

If you can't pay your bills, you feel stressed out. We both know what it's like not to have money. Sally remembers once when she couldn't write her mother a letter because she didn't have money for a first class stamp. Jennifer remembers paying a grocery store in pennies and nickels in order to buy lunch for her daughter. But in every case, every situation, there are choices.

First of all, we learned we could call up a creditor and announce to the company the payment schedule that would work for us. As in, "I will pay you ten dollars a week as soon as my check is in." You can barter for cents on the dollar for debts, taxes and sometimes services. Sally once paid off a $500 pediatrician's bill with wooden toys for the doctor's waiting room (her ex-husband was a woodworker). It's just a matter of looking from a variety of different directions, understanding which Monsters have fed you beliefs that have stopped you from moving forward.

Jennifer lives in a home perched on a ridge with a spectacular view of the mountains, a dream she couldn't have imagined years ago. Sally lives close to the beach in California on her own little piece of heaven, exactly what she has envisioned and chosen for herself.

How did we get from poverty to luxury? By making better choices every day. We went to night classes. We were willing to feel humiliated and ask for help, money, food, whatever it took to get to the next stage. There were whole years we never had a day off, but it was worth it. Why? Because we knew we were getting somewhere. The stress comes from working hard for no good reason.

Dealing with stress doesn't always mean less work. It can just mean giving yourself choices, and not feeling cornered. It can mean understanding there are choices in accepting or rejecting stress or outside pressure.

Stressor Exercise 2

What stresses you out? Often it's the opinions/attitudes of others. A great motto for this is "Who cares?" Make a diary. Note when you feel stressed out, exactly where that stress is coming from. For instance, maybe you hate traffic because you're so powerless when stuck in it. What about bringing along snacks, tapes and CDs, a cell phone and a tape of funny jokes. Change the circumstances *inside* the car because you can't make traffic move faster than it's going.

List what stresses you out:

1. _____

2. _____

3. _____

4. _____

How can I make it fun, or at least palatable? Be creative! What are some options?

1. _____

2. _____

3. _____

4. _____

Stressor Exercise 4

Whose negativity stresses you out? How can you choose to let it go?

1. _____

2. _____

3. _____

Stressor Exercise 5

In order to put stress in perspective, ask yourself:

☞ *Who told you this task was important?*

☞ *What will happen if it doesn't get done?*

☞ *What will I be able to do then?*

☞ *How can I be responsible to the people counting on this?*

☞ *Will this be important five days from now? In five years? How about in five hundred years?*

☞ *What is the picture I have of this when it is completed?*

☞ *Is there another way to get that picture or result?*

☞ *Can I have a part of the picture and could that be enough?*

Ask others in your life:

☞ *What about this expectation is the most important to you?*

☞ *What piece of this can wait?*

☞ *What can we do to meet this need if this doesn't work?*

☞ *Ask others involved how they would solve the problem.*

Facing the Monster Stressor: Our Stories

Sally

"Sorry I'm late," I said to the assembled group. I was totally stressed out about the lack of parking outside the meeting hall. The luncheon guest speaker was talking about—what else? Stress. He dutifully went through the list of all the symptoms of stress: headaches, backaches, nosebleed, hair loss, shoulder pain, dizziness, bleeding gums, indigestion, increase in appetite, decrease in appetite, fatigue, gain or loss of weight, depression and irritability.

I was going through my divorce and asked what I should do if I had all those symptoms one right after the other. The speaker said those were problems that couldn't be addressed in an hour luncheon meeting. Apparently stress that serious was worth at least $90 an hour on a shrink's couch.

What I learned much later was that stress is a matter of choice. All hell can be breaking loose around you, but you can choose to interpret it as interesting, challenging or amus-

ing. In fact, you can shed the panic the way a snake sheds its skin, and still address the very real issues. You just don't have to get hooked.

Jennifer

After two failed marriages, I was so depressed I believed that I'd never have a healthy relationship. As a result, I was a basket case. I remember that time of my life vividly. I was on a television tour and so distraught I had to keep running into the bathroom to put on more makeup before going in front of the cameras, because I kept promptly crying it right back off. It was about this time I picked up a book recommended by a friend, and as I was trying to wade through it (because it was a bit convoluted and a slow read), I happened on a line that blew my socks off: "We create our own reality."

No way! Naturally I thought it had to be a misprint. I mean I couldn't have created two lousy marriages, pain, poverty, and all the other negatives that kept popping up in my life. I tried to ignore it, but again and again I kept thinking, What if there is some truth here? Wouldn't we have incredible power? *That's where my journey began, caught fire and led to the understanding that by learning how to think smarter, more creatively and change the old beliefs, we then have choices in every part of our lives. We have tremendous power we never knew existed.*

Stressor Exercise 5

Write what others have expected from you, and how you can change your attitude.

Stressful expectations from others:

1. _____

2. _____

3. _____

What I choose to do now:

1. _____

2. _____

3. _____

Sally

Ka-runch! "Oh, @#$%*&*!" *I was pulling out of my driveway when one of the stone pillars flanking the entrance jumped out in front of my car and scratched the rear fender. I swear it had nothing to do with my blaring radio and the cute man I was watching mow the lawn across the street. I was about to visit my friend Patty, in Syracuse, New York, and it was a four-hour drive from my home in New Jersey.*

Anyway, I called Patty and told her I couldn't come. I was completely stressed out over getting quotes for bodywork to repair the damage, and having to run all over town to take care of the car. I told her I had to spend my travel money—$300—on fixing my car, and as it was, the bodywork was going to cost me $350.

"Wow," she said, "isn't your car really old?"

Yes, I had to admit it was old, but I told her my father always said you had to fix your car dents right away or else people would think you were dirt-poor trash driving around junk cars.

"Oh, I'm sorry," Patty said. "I thought your father was dead."

"Oh, he is dead," I replied. "He died four years ago."

She said, "Let me see if I have this straight. A man who has been dead four years is telling you to spend $350 on a car whose bluebook value is $200, and for this pearl of wisdom you're going to blow off a great weekend?"

I went to a hardware store, got steel wool and car spray paint, and covered the dent myself so it wouldn't rust. I was packed and on my way to Syracuse the next day. I gave up my father's advice and gave up my stress.

Think of the messages that are still alive and well in your head. Things teachers told you or friends warned you about. Perhaps it's the voice of your deceased grandmother or your first boss or the second-grade teacher who never really liked you.

Jennifer

The amazing thing I remind people of every day in seminars is that we have choices. We don't have to allow stress to get to us unless it's our choice. Now let's go back to the cave days and pretend that a few relatives of ours ran into some prehistoric carnivore; they would've been mighty scared. The blood would rush to their large skeletal muscles in order to allow them to run more effectively and not be that creature's dinner.

Today, if we get frightened because we've been called into our boss's office, or we hear a noise in a darkened room, blood rushes to our large skeletal muscles to help us flee more effectively. If our ancestors picked up clubs to fight one an-

other and protect their home fronts, blood rushed to their hands to enable them to fight. Today if we get so angry we want to throw the phone or a plate of spaghetti at someone, blood rushes to our hands to enable us to fight. Our bodies are reacting the way they did thousands of years ago, but our ability to handle the stress has changed. Without a physical outlet for our adrenaline we can make ourselves sick. But what if we could keep from reacting?

There's a story that Buddha could not be stressed out, that nothing could bother him or destroy his calm. A man who wanted to break through Buddha's meditative state traveled the world until he found Buddha, and then began screaming obscenities at him.

Finally, Buddha turned to the man and asked a simple question: "If someone gives you a gift, and you do not accept it, who does it belong to?"

The man pondered a second and said, "I guess it still belongs to the giver."

"Precisely," Buddha said, "and if you give me obscenities and other negative energy, and I don't accept it, then who does it belong to?"

The man thought a bit longer, got angry and left.

Just because someone gives us a gift of negativity or anger or bad news, just because someone throws something at us, this does not mean we have to accept it or take it. We can refuse it, ignoring the abuse or negativity or bad advice. We can decide it's not the gift for us, thank you anyway.

Sally

The elevator doors opened to the American Festival Café,

*one of the restaurants near the ice rink at Rockefeller Center
in New York City. Flashes from cameras went off everywhere
as a very harried-looking Brooke Shields entered, with press
people reminding the star that she had a very short time at
this particular function. Ms. Shields turned to her audience—more than one hundred children who would return to
a homeless shelter later that evening—who clustered around
her. Her whole manner changed as she sat down on the floor
and read stories to them. She let them move closer, giving completely of herself. If she was stressed by her schedule, not a single child guessed it. She had the ability to be totally giving
and in the moment—a great example for all of us.*

Stressor Exercise 6

Many experts on stress agree that deep breathing and relax-
ation, while very simplistic, are the keys to dealing effectively with much of the aggravation we encounter on a daily
basis. Try this: sit back in a chair and relax. Unfold your
arms and legs, feet flat on the floor. Breathe deeply, exhale
slowly. Picture yourself on a beautiful island you've been to,
or your fantasy vacation spot. Listen to the birds, see the
clouds, hear the waves. Smell the honeysuckle and feel the
breeze on your face. Let your mind go on a break. Do this
for at least five minutes; it's a mini-recess that rejuvenates
and energizes.

Stressor Exercise 7

Find out where the pressure is coming from and send it
back. Ask Who is stressing you out? What is stressing you
out? Money, work, tests, relationships, time constraints,

neighbors, relatives? Whatever it is, you have a choice. Either accept all that comes with your current plan, and work on getting organized or share the work so you're less stressed.

You can also change your priorities and diminish the amount of work you have to produce. What are your expectations? Do you overestimate what can be accomplished? Can you let go of other tasks, priorities, goals?

If you're stressed out by others you must choose whether you'll leave or stay. If you stay, you must decide what your boundaries are, list them, communicate them and stick to them.

If it's a child that's stressing you out, try asking other parents for support. If it's your parents who're stressing you out, work with other people your age for support. When it comes to making a plan to end stress, you must be very clear in which ways you're choosing that stress instead of really coping with situations—while all the time you're convinced others are causing the stress. State your objective. List the steps you need to take to get there. No, we don't mean put a contract on the obnoxious neighbor, but you could refuse to acknowledge his or her wisecracks.

Give your mind and body a break, a recess, in order to go back and handle the stress from a more rational perspective. What do you already do that enables you to leave your stress at the door, and is healthy for you? Garden, clean house, race motorcycles, crochet, read, meditate, walk, walk a dog, play the piano, shop, sing? Only you know what's already built in as a fail-safe mechanism to help you handle the stress going on around you. Use it to your advantage. Ask yourself:

☞ *"What am I doing to create my stress in this situation?"*

☞ *"What do I believe I have to do or take that may not be mine to accept?"*

☞ *"What is the lesson?"*

☞ *"How can I be sure not to repeat this?"*

Stressor Exercise 8

Copping out or taking control? List your responsibility for taking on stress from others. Have you said any of these things today?

You made me_____

I couldn't, because you_____

I can't_____

because you won't let me.

You allow yourself to be affected by others because you care what they think. If you're involved with someone who really does control you by threatening harm to you or others, please seek help from social services. People who threaten are dangerous and to be taken seriously, not given a second chance. If the person is dangerous—meaning they can hurt you and ones you love—you must get out. You must seek help.

Sometimes, we're just surrounded by people with very negative speech patterns. They may not even know they're negative because they grew up in a negative household, and it doesn't seem all that bad to them. In fact, they think you're way too sensitive if you're being pulled down by negative speech. You have a right to set a boundary which requests that negative talk and negative responses not be shared. For a while they won't have much to say, until they relearn a kinder way to talk. But we can assure you, most people know how to speak politely. If they didn't, they'd never get served at a restaurant, get into a movie or get their plumbing fixed.

If you're afraid of someone being angry with you, you'll have to be willing for them to be in a snit for a while. That's the only way you can have your life back. You may even ask them why having your wishes respected threatens them. Remember the *Monster Lies* tell you life is a popularity contest, that everyone has to love you or there's something wrong with you. Think just how wrong this statement is. When you reflect on anyone you admire—a political figure, an author, a teacher, a professional, the coach of a winning team—you'll realize immediately how many times they disagree. They say *no,* and refuse to do everything others want them to do. Life is definitely not a popularity contest. Now go out and do something for yourself. You deserve it.

Stressor Exercise 9

Draw a picture of something that causes you stress: Now color it funny colors. Put it in the copier and make it really small or really big. Stick play-putty over it and stretch it into weird shapes. Take the picture, tear it in tiny, pieces, blow

---

them away. Remember, you have the ability to play this issue up or to make it behave and act sensibly. You have the right to tell your boss that, as much as you want to be a team player, you can't be the whole team and do in one afternoon a job that takes four people three days—even if she really, really needs it!

Stressor Exercise 10

Find ways to cope effectively with your stress. What works best for you?

✓ Surround yourself with colorful posters, flowers, soothing music.

✓ Enter pleasant sayings in your Day Timer.

✓ Put photos of people you care about in sight.

Ask yourself how to stay cool around a problem and then re-design it. Example: Missed a flight? Can you have a conference call?

✓ Forgot to take the dog to the vet? Can a neighbor help?

✓ Messed up your PowerPoint presentation? Can you get your audience to talk about their biggest need, their biggest success?

Write five things you can do to deal with specific recurring stressful events:

1._____

2. _____

3. _____

4. _____

5. _____

Reminders

Stress robs you of your peace, purpose and happiness, because it doesn't allow you to be happy in the moment. As long as you're tense and pushing to meet the next deadline, you'll never enjoy life as you go, and then it will be gone.

Actress Lana Turner had a great deal of trauma and pain in her life, and in an interview on A&E Network she was asked how she'd dealt with it all and managed to keep on going. She replied, "Whatever happened yesterday is gone. I have only today."

Today is the only perspective to work from. One of the best things you can tell yourself when stress starts to smother and incapacitate you is: "All energy toward the future. None toward the past." How do you keep the energy focused on the future? You build up your stress reduction muscles.

Your Action Plan

List all the stresses you feel.
1. Determine which locations seem the most stressful.
    in the shower
    in bed
    at the dinner table
    stuck in traffic

at work
at school
other_____

2. Determine which part of the day is worse.
first thing
before lunch
riding home
other_____

3. Determine what day is the most stressful.
Friday afternoon
Monday morning
Sunday morning
other_____

4. Determine which people you feel are pressuring you.
boss
spouse
parent/in-law
professor
neighbor
other_____

5. Determine why one person's expectations are important enough to deplete your health or deprive you of your peace of mind. In life there are few victims and a lot of volunteers.

Make a list of what you're going to do about it and when.

✓ Set achievable goals with your boss.

✓ Talk to your children about acceptable hours.

✓ Talk to your roommates about respecting your privacy.

✓ Request that your spouse stop screaming orders.

✓ Leave half an hour earlier; change hours at work.

✓ What else would you like to do?

✓ If your job stresses you out, what else could you do?

Make a reality check list.
Is the amount of stress proportional to the issue? If not, diminish the stress by informing others that you're not going to buy into the situation any longer. Often just understanding there are options and choices—that you're not locked in, no matter what the perception—will begin to reduce your stress and allow your life to change in ways you've never even dreamed of.

Summary

When you REVEAL the truth about Stressor, you see stress comes from an idea that we should be doing something or managing something we cannot always control. We need to separate out the feeling of pressure and impending disaster from what can be done. Most likely the action we need to take lies in communicating with others what we can and cannot do regarding the situation. Make a choice to let go of what cannot be controlled. After all, if you're stuck in traffic, stressing out will not make the cars move any faster. When you can ACT to control the panic and fear, you'll have more energy to calm down and take charge of the situation—and your life.

Begin today observing all the behavior that has pushed

your stress buttons in the past. Know you get to make conscious choices moment by moment on how you're going to react. You may not be able to control events, but you have the power to choose exactly how you're going to respond to them. Right now, start to weed out what you can't control, choose how you're going to feel (yes, we really get to choose our feelings), and the RESULT is that your stress levels begin to drop.

CHAPTER FIVE
The Monster Lie Perfecto

The truth Perfecto doesn't want you to know:
The only true mistake is the opportunity not taken.

W e're going to REVEAL exactly how this nasty little Monster sabotages your plans and stops you from taking risks. You'll learn how It tricks you into questioning your abilities and strengths. We'll show you how to ACT to regain control, find the freedom to take appropriate risks and get better RESULTS.

Meet the Monster Perfecto

"Step on a crack, you'll break your mother's back." Whoa, not too much pressure there! As children we're given strong messages that perfect grades and perfect behavior—which meant being still and quiet—were good. Low grades and squirming were not good. Grade school was a test to see exactly where on that continuum we would fit, and the *Monster Lie* was that our performance in school would be an indicator of how happy and smart and successful we'd be as adults.

Perfecto is in Its glory at school, but It lives in the office, church and at home as well. Grades and titles are the most important thing to It. Never mind that the way people survive has much more to do with negotiating skills, bargaining, charisma, humor, compassion, style, grace and insight than knowing who the name of the eighteenth President was, the number of Psalms and the capital of Arizona. School rewards children who are linear thinkers. It sets up other children, who learn differently, to feel inadequate or less-than-perfect. If we are those children, we also take this baggage into adulthood.

Not only do we abhor mistakes in our culture, we hold out great honor only to those who do it "right," by which we mean those who conform to the expectations of society and reflect our own view of the world. We don't necessarily mean those who are able to solve problems or who are happy.

Being right is not always the same thing as being smart. Why? Because when we have to do everything right, we can never let our guard down, never relax, never be honest. After all, we're already supposed to be doing it perfectly. We also can't take the risks needed for breakthroughs and innovations. Yet, if our competitors aren't afraid of risks and can afford even a few calculated mistakes, they'll mop us up in the marketplace.

Mistakes are often trips down alternative roads. It's not always necessary for the road to even join up with the main highway. Some side trips teach you things about the direction you should be heading later on. "Travel broadens the mind." All trips are learning experiences. Even if we return to the main road covered in mud and bug bites!

Perfecto's Voice

Perfecto's voice is shrill and condescending. It takes on a pompous I-told-you-so tone:

You ought to be ashamed of yourself.
You know better than that.

At your age and you can't even . . . .
How can you be so stupid?
Everyone understands this.
This is child's play—get with it, and hurry up.
I thought you were smarter than that.
Any idiot can do this with his eyes closed.
What's the matter with you?
Geez, just watch me again. This is so easy.
You're not trying; you're just not trying.

Perfecto Exercise 1

How does Perfecto belittle you for not being perfect? Whose voice is speaking the loudest?

Example:

Perfecto's words: *You can't get any of these problems*
Who said that?   *Mrs. Black, math teacher.*

Perfecto's words:_____

Who said that?_____

Perfecto's words:_____

Who said that?_____

Perfecto's words:_____

Who said that?_____

Visualizing Perfecto

Perfecto is a little package of precision. Its close-clipped fur is always just-groomed. It wears a bow tie that is always straight and glasses that are never smudged. It's hell-bent on catching you in the act of not being perfect. It looms in hallways and sits in the back seat of your car. Nothing in your life goes unjudged. Perfecto never compliments you on the things you do correctly because it's expected of you. But It always reminds you that you're on the brink of disaster when you mess up.

Beware of Perfecto's twisted logic. If you don't, you might take It seriously, and that could hurt you very deeply. You could begin to suspect that Perfecto has a point. But It doesn't have a point. It is wrong, wrong, wrong. See Perfecto as a little twit with a nasty disposition.

How Does Perfecto Limit You?

It's so easy to feel stupid or inadequate or worthless if you make mistakes. The voice of Perfecto has spoken to us since someone first laughed at our effort to draw, walk, or talk. Everyone remembers being a child and feeling humiliated in front of others for being wrong or different. This has been indelibly imprinted in our thinking. Then our shame can become almost a reflex action against progress.

Perfecto doesn't believe you should be allowed a learning curve to do new things. Mistakes make you bad; perfection makes you good. It loves elementary school when only the children who can memorize answers perfectly get stars. It forgets that all innovation in science comes from trial and error. In fact, scientists talk about finding a "probable" match. They scan data on a computer searching for answers. The computer tries to fit pieces of data together and might scan 100,000 choices before it finds a match. That means there were

999,999 non-matches or "mistakes." Scientists spend a lot of time eliminating non-matches; they're often as eager to identify what doesn't work as what does, because that's important information. Knowing what doesn't work tells them much more about what will work and why.

Facing the Monster Perfecto: Our Stories

Sally

I'm trying to learn to snow board. I'm an expert skier, so the thought of spending hours on the bunny slope is excruciating. Not only that, but I have developed a style when I ski that's fluid and controlled and graceful and sophisticated. When I snow board the opposite adjectives apply. I'm awkward, nerdy, pathetic and jerky, and I sit in the snow a lot (that is when I am not eating it in a face plant). In fact, the only plus I've found in snow boarding is that if you have to walk down the hill a snow board is easier to carry than two skis and two poles.

One of the reasons I hate the learning process is that I pride myself on looking good. I don't look good on a snowboard. When I was forced to learn new things in grammar school, such as math or history, I remember thinking I couldn't wait to be a grownup so I would never have to be humiliated in front of a group of my peers again. Mistakes and ridicule go hand in hand.

Jennifer

The problem is, people buy into the belief that we have to look good right up front, no learning curve allowed. I take

103

jazz classes, and from time to time I bring along a new friend to these classes. While they're not for basic beginners, anyone is welcome to come and do what they can. Interestingly, some people I've brought immediately learn and get in a little exercise. Others feel foolish and leave.

Author and Aikido master George Leonard, in his book Mastery *talks about the necessity of looking foolish in order to go forward. Even if we tamed down the word foolish to "less than perfect," it still paralyzes many people from moving forward.*

A friend of mine once signed up for a class in French. Now, this person is a very successful executive, used to having things her own way. She stayed in the class only about two weeks, but no one who knew her well was surprised. Getting thrown into a situation where she not only didn't know the answers, but could risk looking foolish in the process, was more than she could bear.

When I talk to junior and senior high students, I tell them how important it is to make mistakes—lots and lots of them. How can you ever expect to get where you want to be unless you're willing to go out and ask, try and learn?

Sally and I keep learning, therefore, we keep making mistakes. But no one is keeping track, thank goodness. The way I figure, the more mistakes I make now, the more I'm accelerating my progress. If I have to make mistakes in order to learn and grow and develop, let them happen!

When we grow up, we spend huge amounts of energy trying to avoid making mistakes, or being caught in our mistakes. We avoid stretching too far out of our comfort zone. Why? Because there's never been a reward for making mistakes. We've been so conditioned that mistakes are bad and make us look bad, it's a wonder that anyone takes a risk. Some personalities are more risk-takers than others, but failing is not an easy thing to cope with. All our messages in school and in sports focus on being number one; nobody remembers number two.

Sally

I met Ms. Jayne Meadows at a celebrity event just as I was finishing my manuscript for The Baby Boomer's Guide to Menopause. *Knowing her excellent work with Steve Allen, portraying great women in history on the television show* Meeting of the Minds, *I thought her name would be great for a quote on the back of my book. I was so excited when I called her agent, my brain skipped a gear, and I asked to speak with Audrey Meadows—Alice on the* Honeymooners *television show—who died years ago. The voice on the other end of the phone said "Ms. Meadows is deceased." Stunned that someone I'd just met days before had died, it took me a minute to realize my mistake. Sheepishly, I redialed and asked for Jayne Meadows. Ms. Meadows graciously agreed to give me a quote. I e-mailed her to verify the quote. This time I misspelled her name—Jane Meadows! However she still graciously returned the quote with the correct spelling of her name.*

One thing you learn in business is, don't get someone's name wrong. I think you can add here: don't confuse that person with someone who's dead. I could have let my mistake make me crawl under a rock, but instead, I sent back a thank-you note. Jayne Meadows is a very forgiving, kind and classy lady.

Perfecto Exercise 2

What are you afraid of trying because it may make you look bad? What did you try once and give up because you weren't the best at it? List three things you'd like to do if you could be perfect at each of them right away:

1. _____

2. _____

3. _____

Would you try any of these if you could make mistakes, but still be good at them eventually? If not, why not?

Being accomplished in life means we must be willing to look bad for a while, which is often the hardest thing to do. Children of alcoholics or emotionally unstable adults have an even harder time. If they err, their lives are often threatened. The stakes for perfection are very high. The rules always change so the children never know what is perfect and what is a mistake. Often they get punished one day for something that was acceptable the day before.

Perfecto wants to stop us from succeeding by making us afraid to do the one thing that separates people of accomplishment from people with a bunch of good ideas . . . taking risks. Perfecto wants you to stop trying out all the options until you find the key to your success. Be forewarned that not everyone will approve of your making mistakes. They'll try to save you the embarrassment by telling you how to do something. They'll warn you, and they won't be there to support you when you make the real Grandfather of all mistakes. But, so what? Evaluate their warnings and weigh the risks before you make a decision. If you wait for approval from your boss, spouse, mother, fiancé, teacher, friend or mentor, you'll live a life of anticipation and disappointments. You, on the other hand, are the most influential person you know.

Reward yourself for trying, and let the outcome take care of itself. Just look at what we lose, what we fail to learn, and what message we pass on to employees, children, friends and associates. People learn from being led, not told, and when we set criteria that says don't question, risk or take any chances, it's no surprise that we don't get what we need from these people. They're too afraid of saying the wrong thing, thus blocking the creative thinking needed for the process.

Perfecto Exercise 3

What's the "Best Mistake" you ever made? Often in life we make unpopular decisions. We go to a small unknown college instead of an Ivy League school. We go into the ministry instead of computer technology. We start a store in a neighborhood that already has five stores of the same type. We marry outside the family expectations. We have children early, late or not at all. And guess what? It was the best thing we ever did.

Now list all the decisions that you made that were considered mistakes by others and turned out for the best.

1. _____

2. _____

3. _____

4. _____

Reread this list on a regular basis. This is your confirmation that "mistakes" can be good. The smart thinker learns what is possible and realizes that those giving advice probably gave up on their own dreams years ago. Continuing in the face of rejection, in the face of mistakes, is what steers a person in the right—and often new—direction.

Perfecto Exercise 4:
How long does it take?

Have you ever learned a musical instrument? How about a new sport? Did you ever learn a foreign language? How long did it take? Some things take ten days to learn, and ten years to be really good at it. Why then, do we beat ourselves up when we have to struggle to learn new things? Computers, new jobs, VCRs, dancing, parenting. We get totally stressed out when we have to learn. Don't we know there'll be some failures and false starts? We all hate looking bad.

Write down three things you had to learn in the last five years, and how long it took to learn them.

1._____

2._____

3._____

How long should it take to learn new things? Here's the key to understanding adult learning curves: it takes as long as it takes. When you were in grammar school and the teacher was trying to instruct twenty kids Spanish all at the same time, she had to decide how long each section of the curriculum would take. She had to make up an average learning time. Some will be advanced and some will be behind. None of that has to do with how people learn. You'll learn tennis or Spanish or computer programming or how to drive a car in as much time as it takes you. In fact, educators say you should expect to have some new idea repeated 7-20 times before you remember it. That is a long time, and it may be more if you don't have a reference point—that is, if it's not similar to something you already know.

There's no right or wrong learning curve length unless you choose to listen to those people who're setting your standards for you. If you want to speed up your learning curve, then do what every famous athlete has done for centuries: Hire a coach. Or if you can't afford a coach, or don't have time to be tutored, then read about how other people accomplished similar goals.

Perfecto Exercise 5

Find three experts, or at least three individuals who do something very well. Ask each of these people how long it took to master what they do, and what were the biggest mistakes they made during the learning process. Explain you're asking because you're changing your core philosophies on learning, and you're looking for inspiration. You'll be amazed at what you hear.

Example:

Expert:	*Magician*
Mistakes they made:	*Fell off stage during a show.*

Expert:_____

Mistakes they made:_____

Expert:_____

Mistakes they made:_____

Expert:_____

Mistakes they made:_____

Jennifer

A friend of mine told me once that if I put something out there—begin talking about it—that idea will eventually become a reality. I thought about it and I tried it. This has been a technique I've used again and again to achieve what I want. I begin by talking about something as if it's a definite reality waiting to happen. Then little by little—and sometimes not so slowly—it does become a reality. This is not wishful thinking. It's the awareness that what we think about expands. If we think fear and failure when we try something—Bingo—that's what we get.

A great way to look at shortening your learning curve—making those essential mistakes and getting on with the learning and accomplishing—is to remember that for most things, if one person has done it, many others can do it, too. It's just learning the model he or she used to do it or learn it.

I was having terrible trouble learning to wear contact lenses. Everything in the world was happening except getting the contact into my eye. Then a friend left a message of encouragement on my answering machine, stating simply that if she could learn to wear contacts, anyone could learn.

On the tennis court, a dynamite partner of mine who has graceful strokes and a powerful serve, said her first coach had given up on her. Again, if she could learn to serve, anyone could.

Use this piece of knowledge. All the experts had to make lots and lots of mistakes to become the experts. They knew if someone else could do it, they could do it, too. They were willing to learn from someone who had already mastered what they needed, and were willing to make the prerequisite mistakes to get there.

Sally

Write a song about how it feels to fail and then discuss where those feelings come from. My kids and I used to sing the "Sad, Mad, Bad Day" song when we had one of those days. We each got a chance to make up verses, and then we'd sing the song until we'd be giggling hysterically. Do you expect to be perfect sooner than others—and if so, why? Why should you escape the learning curve?
(This is perfect for Delta Blues or Country style)
I tried to get a job doing health care work
The lady said go away; I was a big jerk.
So I went to the hospital and tried there.
They put me in the emergency room and transplanted my hair.

(It helps to get silly!)
I got the I'm Bad-Bald-and-Broke Blues.

Making fun of your own pain is a first step to achieving power and overcoming this *Monster Lie* Perfecto, who wants us to feel so awful that we stop aiming for our dreams. Comics make a lot of money by poking fun at their pain. There's even a group called Comedians in Recovery, stand-up comics who, having overcome addictions, now go around performing for people in rehabilitation programs. They give a very strong message that pain is a part of the learning curve of life. It's a process we all go through.

Perfecto Exercise 6

What do you want so much that you're willing to be wrong and make lots of mistakes—or even have a thousand mismatches before you get it right? Where can you give yourself permission to be wrong—possibly very wrong? List those who'll likely ridicule you on this, and why you should care about their opinions. When can you let go of the need to prove and define yourself by others' standards? That's when you can relax and begin doing and having the things that are important to you.

Perfecto Exercise 7

Decide right now how much you're willing to take in rejection and setbacks before you call it quits. How much money are you willing to spend? How many mistakes are you willing to make? How much time will you invest?

Project:_____

Time frame:_____

Money:_____

Irritation:_____

Reputation:_____

Then what? List all the things you're afraid of when you think about making mistakes. Example: *I'll be embarrassed*. List what you'll do then: Keep asking, "Then what?"

Forgiving others and yourself is an important first step toward taming Perfecto. But by "forgive" we mean accept that you must go on and not hold on to the hurt and anger. This is not to say you approve of the person who hurt you or harmed you in any way, but in order to move forward and put your energy where it needs to be. It is essential to let it go. Remember, there are many people who live in fear and anger. This is their choice, not yours. Their negativity cannot harm you unless you allow it.

Perfecto Exercise 8

Imagine you're in a huge auditorium. This might be a sports stadium, a civic center, a performing arts arena, but it's huge. Now think of all the people you're still angry at over some wrong they've done to you. Perhaps they discouraged your progress, pointed out your failures, warned you not to try because you'll only screw it up, told you to forget it and stop while you're ahead—you're lucky you got this far.

Put those charming souls in your auditorium, front row. See how many people you're still wasting your precious energy on. Look at them up close, scrutinize them, how arrogant they look, how angry they might appear, how pathetic they really are in trying to frighten you into submission. Can you see through their façades? Maybe yes, maybe no.

113

Now decide you're going to put your energy to better use from now on, and let go of any and all anger you have toward these people. Bless them, feel kindness, or at the very least, know they're not worth using your energy on any more. Let any anger go. If your memory brings them up again in the future, just softly say, "No more. He's not worth it" and get on with your great life. If you dwell on these folks they get to hurt you again. Why give them that power?

By the way, we both did this exercise, and our greatest shock was how many people were sitting in our auditoriums. There were old girl friends and ex-wives of our boyfriends and husbands, ex-bosses and confrontational associates. Between us we could have supplied enough extras for an elaborate movie production!

What if it's yourself you can't forgive? Try remembering the rest of your life has some purpose, and you can't effectively move forward if you're dragging around all the disappointments and sins from your past. Again, all the energy toward the future, none toward the past. You can only control and produce in the present, and plan for the future. The past is dead air; walk away from it.

Perfecto Exercise 9

Where can you speak up right now, beginning today? Think of three places where you would like to voice an opinion, or ask a question, make a comment, learn more about a procedure, but you knew you couldn't ask or communicate as succinctly, as "perfectly" as you should, and so you said nothing. Then go out and speak up . . . it's amazing how much less perfect you have to be when you're getting the information you need, and learning what you want to know. Don't be afraid to write your questions or statements down on three-by-five cards. Jennifer and Sally are top speakers, and they still use notes as reminders! Hint: they call them agendas.

Name three places where you can have a voice:

Place	_Date_
1.	
2.	
3.	

If you've been surrounded by Perfecto, it's time to start making some mistakes, take a learning curve, be willing to look imperfect in the eyes of perfectionists and get ready for more success, fun and results in your life. When people are afraid to make mistakes at work several things happen. First of all, nobody wants to take responsibility for anything, so everybody passes the buck. Another thing that happens is that everybody does everything the same old way, until the company folds or the employees die of boredom. You can't stay ahead of the competition by playing it safe.

How do you take the sting out of being wrong or messing up? You practice allowing yourself to be wrong. You learn how to find the gift in the goof!

Perfecto Exercise 10

"Argue for your limitations, and you get to keep them," said author Richard Bach. Yet these little voices in our head are

SALLY FRANZ & JENNIFER WEBB

often our most subtle saboteurs, reminding us consistently of the errors we make or might make or could make if we're not really careful. Both of us are aware how often we're hearing their reminders:

> *You'll never make it in that parking spot. You never parallel park well.*
> *Forget trying to work out in the morning. You know you don't have the discipline to do it three times a week.*
> *Get used to that golf swing. You'll never be able to do it any better. If you could, you'd have improved by now.*

Now what are your voices? List three Lies you tell yourself and who told you to believe them. Example: "You can never get in that spot. You've never been good at parallel parking." Was this your driving instructor who hated his job and told everyone to improve? A boyfriend who thought he was Mario Andretti and said no one, especially girls, could drive like him? A husband or a mother? Who crowned you as the "poorest driver of the Twenty-first century?" If you still think you need help, take a driving course. Then get your diploma and give out copies. We hope you get the message that most of your "carved-in-stone" opinions about yourself are actually written in sand, and can crumble quite easily when examined.

Belief:_____

Person responsible:_____

Belief:_____

Person responsible:_____

116

Belief:_____

Person responsible:_____

The past only has power to destroy your future if you keep resurrecting it. No one will ever know all the reasons why things happened the way they did. But Perfecto has you by the throat if you obsess on the past, because that will prevent you from living in the present. Mistakes and tragedy happen. Most of the time we aren't even aware of the tragedies others have let go of. We only know about their old baggage if they keep unpacking it in front of you.

Reminders

A Mistake is a Moment that Vanishes.

A young piano player who worked at a hotel in Tulsa, Oklahoma said she loved live performances. When asked why, she said, "Well, if you make a mistake, the wrong note hangs in history but for a moment in time, and then it is gone." She also loved it that there was no memory of the note, it had simply passed like a bird in flight. What a great thought! A mistake is a moment in time that vanishes like sound.

Your Action Plan

Here's something you can do immediately. Decide what you would do right now if:

☞ You were twenty again (or if you're twenty, then ten or fifteen).

☞ Failure was not an option. You would have all the knowledge, support or resources to succeed.

☞ No one would judge your progress.

Remember, according to research, the number one emotion people feel on their deathbeds is regret. Regret for not doing more of what they loved, for not trying what they dared not do, and for not finding the time to live in the moment.

Make a pact with yourself that you'll decide on one goal. List it here. Plan the first five steps you'll take. List the date when each one will be accomplished; remember to make them a series of small successes. Start the first one today, within the next six hours if possible.

What I want is:_____

On a scale of 1 (not much) to 10 (want it a whole lot) rate your desire:_____

What it may cost: $_____

How long it might take:_____ (days, months years*).

Number of mistakes, failures, and setbacks I am willing to face:_____

My target completion date is (time, day, month, and year):

_____

Who can help me:

_____

What others have done in a similar situation is:

_____

(* Note: you'll use up the same number of days, months and years whether you start your project or whine about how hard it'll be. So you might as well start now.)

Summary

We've REVEALED that Perfecto paralyzes you, stops your growth and denies you the life you deserve. It's the ubiquitous voice warning you to do it right, or don't do it at all. How do we ACT immediately to get control over Perfecto? Awareness is everything. Remember why you're stuck. It's the cacophony of voices reminding you what would happen, and you've taken them as reality. Look at the Action Plan and decide what you're willing to risk, what will you dare to do regardless of the outcome? Even if you start small, if you do something right away—within the next twenty-four hours—you will begin to see RESULTS almost immediately.

CHAPTER SIX

The Monster Lie Scarcity

The truth Scarcity doesn't want you to know:
The more you hoard, the less you have.

We're going to REVEAL how this Monster traps you into believing you'll never have enough, never have what you really need. It's the voice of fear, the voice that stops you from enjoying what you have and keeps you living in a perpetual state of worry and concern. Now it's time to ACT. We'll give you some practical steps to immediately see RESULTS for abundance in every part of your life.

Meet the Monster Scarcity

Both of us speak from firsthand experience when it comes to Scarcity. Not only have we both been very poor, but as we've accumulated more financial security, we've often felt Scarcity breathing down our backs, hitting us in the soft underbelly with a little thought, "What if all this is short-lived. Then what will you do?"

Scarcity's Voice

Scarcity whispers in your ear with a sound like clawing and scratching and howling. It evokes a picture of every starving child, and a flashback to everything you were told as a young-ster to frighten you into eating your food (children starving in _____) or into working hard so you would not end up penniless and on the streets. You know the voice of Scarcity too well. It is the voice of fear. It is living out of survival instead of generosity.

Well, you're going to pay for all those good times now!
All that money you had was a fluke; now you're going to be poor.
Only rich people can have luxuries; you have to take seconds.
No one owes you a living, young lady.
They're only hiring young / experienced / college educated. You'll never get a job.
You're overqualified. You're underqualified.
You'll have to settle for what you can get.
If they downsize, you'll be out. You'll miss your mortgage payments and be on the streets.
You're going to have to work hard for everything you get in this life.
You're all alone, and nobody is going to help you.
How will you survive? You can't make enough money!
You'll lose everything!
You'll never get out of debt.

The Monster Scarcity wants you to believe survival is based on hoarding, cheating and beating out everyone else. It wants you to buy into a mentality that suggests if you have it, you won't for long—so hold tight.

Scarcity Exercise 1

What does Scarcity whisper in *your* ear? How does this

Monster drive you into fear and panic? List the things Scarcity warns you about on a daily basis. You may have to listen very closely because Its words sound sincere and logical instead of paranoid and frightened.

1._____

2._____

3._____

4._____

5._____

Visualizing Scarcity

Imagine a skeleton with hollow, empty eyes, clutching, bony hands; and clenched teeth. Scarcity believes that hoarding is the only way to protect yourself. Sharing could be suicide. Scarcity is selfish, opportunistic and defensive. It lives in fear and so brings the worst on Itself. It's so busy protecting Itself from being taken advantage of that Scarcity misses opportunities for both Itself and others.

Scarcity believes in a world of limited resources, and for It, this is a reality. It'll tell you there's a limited amount of everything on the planet; just so much energy, food, love, forgiveness, sympathy, good luck, friendship. There is scarcity everywhere. Therefore, you will want to be jealous if others have good things. You will want to horde what you have, and never, never relax or celebrate in your good fortune—because that will jinx it. Scarcity's philosophy: happiness is scarce, love is limited, and good times have a short shelf life.

How Does Scarcity Limit You?

Because we're creatures of habit, and if we've grown up accustomed to scraping together just enough—or if we have everything we need but can't imagine a life of luxury—we've locked this in as our reality, and, therefore, it is. Scarcity feeds off this concept, and reinforces all our worst fears. If we worry constantly about making ends meet with the next paycheck—or paying the student loan off or putting a child through college—we will always have what we're focusing on. It's a self-fulfilling prophecy. Scarcity tells us if something has been one way so far, inevitably that's the only way it can be. This would mean the rich get richer and the poor stay poor. This can often be the case simply because of how they're thinking, where they're putting their energy or worry.

For instance, if you grew up scraping enough together to make car payments or school lunch money, it's hard to relax and allow yourself the pleasure—if not luxury—of feeling financially safe, even if you have a couple of hundred thousand dollars in your savings account. After all, what if the bank fails and you're on the street? Old habits die hard, and old beliefs die even harder.

It's what we focus on that expands. If we focus on poverty, we get more poverty.

Facing the Monster Scarcity: Our Stories

Jennifer

In my seminars, I show a picture of mountains that look very similar to the Rockies, and in the foreground, one can see trash cans with rats scurrying back and forth. When

SALLY FRANZ & JENNIFER WEBB

I asked participants what they see, the answers are a bit like an inkblot test. Some see the beauty, reminisce on a honeymoon in the Rockies or a skiing trip, others talk of the decay and filth in the world today, and how sad it is that Mother Earth is becoming so polluted.

What we focus on expands, whether that focus is on trash or beauty, wealth or poverty. We have much more control than we realize.

Examine what is real about your economic status, and what is being fed to you by the Monster Scarcity. Put your wealth in perspective. Do you have what's really valuable and important to you, such as your family's health and love? Granted, paying bills and living without constant worry and stress is important, but how many thousands of dollars would you take for the life of your parent, significant other, spouse or child? How much money would you take for your eyesight, your health, your sense of humor? We're all blessed in many ways that we forget to acknowledge. Wealth also starts with being grateful for what we've already got.

Why can't you make more money, live in the style you like, help your daughter or mother, take the vacation you've dreamed of? It begins with setting your goal, your ideal salary or the amount of money you want in the bank, and then using a variety of techniques to trick your brain into believing you already possess what you want.

The strange thing about our subconscious, it doesn't always know whether we already have what we're acting as if we've got, or whether we're just pretending. In the same way, our heart beats faster, adrenaline pumps, and we can feel threatened and terrified when we see the knife poised in the air behind the heroine, and all we're doing is sitting quietly in a movie theater watching a thriller—far away from harm.

Taking a cue from accelerated learning techniques, using all your intelligence areas—linguistic, logical, musical, kinesthetic, visual—apply all the learning styles to keep this image of financial security firmly planted in your mind. Smell what it feels like to live where you want. See yourself writing a check nonchalantly. Hear how a new car sounds as it backs out of your driveway. Imagine being out of debt and paying off your credit cards monthly.

Sally

Scarcity shows up in our lives when we feel as if what we have is being threatened. As a Baby Boomer, I remember when the neighborhood rage was building bomb shelters in basements. My father got huge cinderblocks and created a room within a room. He left a window, which I guess could be cemented up if need be. This was to protect us against the likelihood of an atomic bomb attack.

I remember when we asked about it. The idea was that we would all crawl downstairs and live together off canned goods for a few years until it was safe to crawl outside in the glowing embers of the Planet Earth. I pictured the family trip to the lake, five kids in a station wagon for five hours, and then extended the trip to three years with no Howard Johnson's breaks. We would no doubt kill one another within a few weeks!

I also remember being told not to blab it around that we even had a bomb shelter. I had dreams of the neighbors clawing the edges of our house begging to get in, and hearing their agonizing moans as they died slow gruesome deaths. Survival is important, and I suppose that it goes to the fittest. But it sure doesn't do much for trust and community.

The hope is that people have learned enough to work side by side with their neighbors and work together in a crisis.

There are many references in our book to the powers of visualization, of utilizing all your senses, all your learning styles. Affirmations said out loud, or written on a constant basis—we recommend fifteen times a day—are also powerful. We know a well-respected professional speaker, Glenna Salisbury, who swears she got everything she wanted in her life: her husband, the home in the specific location, the jewelry—everything—by cutting out pictures from magazines, pasting very specific images into a collage and pinning this above her desk and dwelling on it to the point of obsession. She says she can't swear exactly how it works, but she got what she wanted. We think she cued her brain to look for what she wanted among all the possibilities that passed by her each day.

Work from the expectancy mode, not the "I'll believe it when I see it" mode. If you ask God for something, pray with the expectancy of results. See the direction you're going and the financial security you want with the expectancy that you'll get it. Otherwise, you'll spend your time holding tightly on to what you've got, hoarding more and ending up with less.

When you say or write your affirmations, are you doing them because you're going to prove to yourself they really won't help? If you don't expect something, you won't be disappointed. If you want to receive what you're focusing on, expect the results you want, and truly understand that you deserve to get them. No one ever did any good in the world by thinking poor, or accepting substandard things. You deserve to have everything you want and more. Then remember it's yours to spread around. Keep your hands open, not clutched. All gifts are for enjoyment—but also to share with others.

Remember, the root of all evil is the "love" of money. That is, using money as a security blanket or a way to control people. If you love money, you will become a slave to it, in debt and never having enough. Money is not a friend. It is a tool to help others and yourself. Ignoring the needs of the world and trying to validate your own soul with money don't work. Using poverty the same way doesn't work either. It's not about the money. It's about taking care of yourself and others. Money is to be used to share, care, heal and celebrate. Whether you're poor or rich, if money runs you, then you will be at its mercy. But if you give freely, without fear of your next meal or protecting your lovely things, you will be happy and money will not control you. Remember this rule: Relationships before bank accounts.

Scarcity Exercise 2

Imagine you're out in your backyard—or park or neighbor's back yard if you don't have one—and you're watering a garden. You're walking with the hose and suddenly the water stops. You turn around to see what's happened, and then it dawns on you, your foot is on the hose. When you take it off—magic!—water again. This happens in our lives, but the foot is our mental attitude of scarcity. We're our own worst enemy. We stop ourselves from having what we need and deserve because we're so sure we can't have it.

Could your salary double this year? If you said a quick and resounding *no,* then why not? Are you worth double the money? If you feel you're not, examine what led you to this assumption. You have to believe you're worth the money or honor or happiness, or you won't allow yourself to have it. Is

127

anyone else you know making more money than they "deserve"? How did they do that? Now list five beliefs you have about what you're not entitled to have, and why. Then go back and find the Lie in those beliefs.

What are your beliefs that might be Lies?

Example:
Belief: I could never own a home
Lie: I have to settle for renting forever.

Belief:_____

Lie:_____

Belief:_____

Lie:_____

Belief:_____

Lie:_____

Belief:_____

Lie:_____

Belief:_____

Lie:_____

Have you seen the car commercial that asks, "Do wealthy people have a right to have safer cars with more air bags and more safety features?" It's explaining a moderately priced vehicle that has the safety features of luxury cars. If you know you have worth, no matter what your financial status, then you're free to let go of worrying about money because you know two things:

1. Financial abundance is there, waiting for you to find it. It's the result of taking financial responsibility—get out of debt, save regularly, stop impulse-buying.
2. How much you have is not a measurement of your worth. You can feel wealthy without any money, or broke and worthless with a million dollars. An attitude of how good you feel, how happy you are is a choice!

What if you gave money to people without expectations? What if you never lent money but just gave it away? So much of our giving has control written all over it. Sharing has a very liberating effect on us. It's reminding us that the more we give of our wealth—or knowledge, time, etc.—the more it keeps flowing back. It isn't ours to keep, but always to pass on. Now, we're not talking about your thirty-year-old child who refuses to work. We're talking about having an open heart to beggars, the homeless and single mothers. I make it a habit, whenever asked for money for food from a homeless person, to offer to buy them a meal instead—and yes, sometimes eat with them. You'd be amazed at the stories I've heard over a burger.

Scarcity Exercise 3

Give away money. Give a dollar bill to someone every day this week, or the equivalent—a cup of coffee and doughnuts. Don't judge if they need it or not. Tip a waiter an extra dollar, give money to a child or derelict, and just share what you have in the way of joy.

Diary of giving:

Amount:	_Date:_	_Person:_
1.		
2.		
3.		
4.		
5.		
6.		
7.		

How do you feel?

If you withhold giving because you can't trust the big charities, then get involved with the community and give where you can watch your gift in action. The message here is that a generous heart is a healthy heart. A tight, stingy heart is a sick heart, spiritually and probably physically as well. Scarcity will limit your friends. People who would be willing to help you will dwindle down to none. Scarcity will kill you off so gradually that in the end the things you feared most—poverty and loneliness—may come to pass.

When you live in an environment of Scarcity, you spend all your energy trying to protect your possessions. Americans love their "stuff." It makes us feel powerful and in control. But anyone who has ever left late for a vacation because they were mowing the lawn, closing up the house or watering the plants knows the awful truth: we're owned by our stuff.

We all like our things, but if we're holding onto our stuff

out of fear, we might look at how that affects us. If we learn to let go and practice generosity, it will enrich our lives. Now, this only works if we give freely, with no expectations of getting in return, or of having the recipient perform to our liking. Give without strings attached.

Remember the story of the monkey and the cookie jar? Some hunters put a jar of cookies in the jungle. The monkey wanted the cookies. He reached inside the cookie jar and grabbed as many as he could. Then he tried to get his hand out, but he had such a large fistful his hand was stuck. The only way to get his hand free was to loosen his hold on some of the cookies. He wouldn't, and so he remained stuck and was captured.

The Monster Scarcity isn't about money. It's about believing the illusion that there simply isn't enough. This mentality is the surest way not to have what we want. When we let go of hoarding and guarding and holding out, we open ourselves to miracles in every direction.

There are ways to trick your mind into trying new patterns—patterns that can often lead to huge breakthroughs. One way is to understand the law of abundance and realize that even though much of the evidence seems to say the opposite, there is, in essence, more than enough for everyone. We've just been conditioned to believe the contrary. As we've already said, old beliefs die hard. Statistics even show there's enough food on the planet to feed the entire world population, but it seems some people are using up more than their fair share of resources.

We dispel the Scarcity mentality by focusing on what we have, on visualizing what we want and acting as if we have it. In other words, if you're panicked over your bills, try to react with generosity, not fear. If you eat out that week, don't leave the waitress the smallest amount for a tip. Double it instead. See your money as if it were the colorful stuff in Monopoly. We've all played this game at one time or another. If you lost it all to pay for landing on someone's hotel, so what? Putting that same degree of nonchalance on money opens your subconscious up for believing you've got what you're visualizing. It alleviates the fear, and helps make it a reality. Obviously, this isn't a license to spend unwisely—just creatively and generously.

Keep in mind these ideas might seem very strange to you—but what have you got to lose? If the old way you're living your life isn't giving you what you want, then it's time to look for alternate ways. Using the right brain, as in these suggestions, can be a powerful source to get results.

We're not suggesting that you be irresponsible and spend like there's no tomorrow. We're saying don't be cheap with others. Be as generous as you can afford to be. Another way to diffuse the power of Scarcity is by trusting in a power higher than yourself. Both of us believe we must be open to the abundance we believe we deserve, and continue to do what we love to do. There are many ways to stand up to Scarcity once we realize those beliefs—those voices we took as the absolute truth—are whispering Lies about what we can and can't have in this life.

Scarcity Exercise 4

Why do some people have more money? Why do the rich get richer? Why do those who seem to be born under lucky stars continue to be lucky? Because they know how to focus their energy, their thoughts. They absolutely tune out the Lies, the voices that they have also heard along the way, but have chosen to ignore. There's an axiom that says: *If someone can do it, anyone can do it.* So if your wealthy neighbor, your super lucky acquaintance, your rich business associate can focus their energies to have everything they want, why can't you?

Could you put in a contact lens before someone said, "If I can do it, believe me you can learn it, too." It's easier to work on your tennis serve if someone says, "It took me forever, but if I can do it, anyone can." Do you think you could speak on stage in front of five thousand people if your coach hadn't said, "I was so scared, I was paralyzed. If I could learn to speak, anyone can." Get the idea?

Write down five things you'd like to do but believe are impossible for you, and then find out what it would take to do those things. We're not telling you to get out there and try all of them right away. We're asking you to research, get the information, find out what steps it would take. You'll see that there are steps, procedures, answers to challenges—and they may seem impossible. But then you can see what you still need to know and what's lacking in your life. Then you can absolutely change it.

Impossible for me to do:

_____

Steps it would take:

1._____

2._____

3._____

4. _____

5. _____

Scarcity Exercise 5

Pass the Plate.

If you attend a church or synagogue, or wherever you worship, drop five times what you usually do in the offering plate the next time you attend. It will probably feel like budget suicide. Most of us give what's left over. Even if we are used to tithing, dropping a five, or twenty or one hundred-dollar bill is awkward because it is not usually done.

Write a check.

Another option is to double or triple what you normally send to your favorite charity at the end of the month. The ASPCA or a battered women's shelter will be delighted.

Now note how hard it was to give. It can be the exact opposite of impulse buying. You hem and haw and are trying to talk yourself out of an amount much bigger than you usually give. Wouldn't it be grand if you didn't think twice about giving, but had a real fit and broke out into a cold sweat around a two-for-one sale! Imagine how different your credit card problem might be. Remember, charitable giving enriches the soul—and it's tax deductible!

Scarcity Exercise 6

Nothing defeats Scarcity quicker than a constant awareness of what we've got to be grateful for. Each morning when you wake up, say, "I, not events, have the power to make me happy or unhappy today. I can choose which it shall be. Yesterday is dead, tomorrow hasn't arrived yet. I have just one day, today, and I'm going to be happy in it.'" Sometimes it takes a brush with death to make us realize how much we value sunsets, peanut butter, laughter, or just waking up alive.

Make a List of Ten Things You Take for Granted:
Examples: *Eyesight, healthy body, breathing, house, job, family, pets, friends, sun in morning, rain, moonlight*.

1. _____
2. _____
3. _____
4. _____
5. _____
6. _____
7. _____
8. _____
9. _____
10. _____

Scarcity Exercise 7

We take thousands of things for granted, including our own bodily functions. For instance, the brain keeps on directing and the heart keeps right on beating.

Look at your list from Exercise 6. One by one, imagine that these aren't part of your existence. As you start to put things into perspective, imagine it's ten years in the future. What would life be like if these things weren't part of your life?

Now think of five things you worry about that relate to Scarcity, such as:

"Will I get the job after I graduate?"
"What happens if I don't get that promotion?"
"What if tuition/insurance/car payments go up? What will I do?"

1. _____

2. _____

3. _____

4. _____

5. _____

When we start to worry about a scarcity that may or may not happen, we're killing off our ability to move forward and have abundance. If the scarcity does happen, then we'll address the issue. In the meantime, we'll be focusing on what we can do about it today, right now.

Scarcity Exercise 8

Make a list of the things you'd miss if today were your last day on earth.

1._____

2._____

3._____

4._____

5._____

Now make a list of all of the things you would rather keep than exchange for an extra month of life:

_____

This exercise helps us place appropriate value on our belongings and bank accounts. If you start giving things away now, if you start sharing now, how will you be affecting others as well as yourself?

Jennifer

I once had to move out of an apartment in one night, as my wild, drug-crazed ex-landlord harassed me. (I've moved a lot in my time!) You realize things aren't really all that relevant sometimes, and that was one of those times. I left much behind, as I was afraid for my life.

If you had to take one or two cherished items with you as you left a burning house or sinking ship, what would you take? Things are things. Who cares how much you have if you aren't happy, content and fulfilled? Things will not fill those emotional needs no matter how much we try to rationalize that they will. In fact, things can trick you into thinking that you're doing well. If you have enough toys you might not even notice how empty you feel. But a life full of things won't be much comfort when you need a friend.

Scarcity Exercise 9

Throw a party. Celebrate life with people you care about. Whether it's only three people and you have popcorn and colas, or twenty friends who bring their favorite casserole (or you order pizza delivery). Many people don't entertain even close friends because they're ashamed of their homes or what they can't provide for food. If that's true, you need new friends. Good friends will bring food and gather in your home regardless of whether they have to sit on barrels or tires or golden-threaded couches.

Sally

I once held a holiday party for fifty people in a one-room apartment. I got my neighbor to store my bed and dining room table for the night. I decorated the mantelpiece with greens and put a card table in the corner with a big bowl of punch. I invited friends who came from every imaginable walk of life. I invited people I liked who'd been a friend to me at one time or another. It was one of the best parties I ever had. I think some of the guests still think the closet door led to the rest of the apartment. Open up your home and open up your heart.

Sally

My grandmother had the following quote read at her funeral: "All that you can take with you in your cold dead hands are the things you gave away." She must have read that saying early in her life because she was always very generous.

Scarcity Exercise 10

Stanford University once asked the top ten percent of its students to write down all their good qualities and all of their bad qualities, and the ratio was six-to-one. Top students at a top university wrote six pages of negatives for every one page of positives. We're all so conditioned to look at our faults—what we do wrong—and that feeds directly into the Scarcity mindset. If we already are doing so many things badly, we better be sure and hold onto what we've got, because we're not smart enough or educated enough or clever enough to ever do any better or get any more.

Write five things you've done in your life that you're proud of, that affected someone else in a positive way. Doesn't matter how big or small, so long as someone benefitted in the process.

1._____

2._____

3._____

4._____

5._____

Reminders

Thank You, Thank You.

A great way to change the mental habit of Scarcity is to say thanks, or just write a note complimenting someone on a job well done, even if it's a job they get paid to do. Look at those you care deeply about but never take the time to tell, then thank them for being wonderful, for being part of your life.

Hoarding Creates Lack.

If you stop and think about it, hoarding is pretty much what most wars are about. People want what others have. They want a shrine, territory, resources, power or food. So, too, in our battle of life, when we dwell on holding on to everything we've got, we're definitely creating an attitude of lack. When we're in constant fear of losing whatever we're hoarding—information, time, money, love—it stops us from moving forward.

Your Action Plan

The best plan of action to face the fears generated by Scarcity is to share what you have with others. The people we know who have the most trouble with this say things like:

People have taken advantage of me. Never again!
Nobody ever gave me anything.
People will expect more from me.
If I give to others who will take care of me?

Being soft on people doesn't teach them anything.
I work hard for my money. Let others do the same.

These feelings of fear are very real. They come from a sense that what you have won't last. A fear that you're all alone in the world and, therefore, must control everything. Keep in mind: what you focus on expands. Lack will create more lack. Abundant thinking—focusing without fear—will create abundance. Now couple that with the understanding you aren't alone. Look around at all the people who can use a kind word from you. Think of at least one true friend you've had, and you'll remember that you always get back more than you give.

List three reasons you're afraid to give to others.

1. _____

2. _____

3. _____

Now ask yourself this: "If I had a million dollars would I feel this way? If I died tomorrow would I feel this way?"

We're not asking you to give away all your food or the mortgage payment or rent. We're suggesting that you be generous with your discretionary money, your free time and your kind words.

Next, think of all the things you can give away (money, time, kind words, etc.) and spend at least ten minutes doing this every day this week.

What I can give away

✓ _____

✓ _____

Finally, for twenty-four hours, act as if money were no problem. Monitor those voices, those Lies that warn us to be careful, remember what could happen, etc. Do not allow these thoughts to create fear. This will take constant awareness, but the results can be staggering. Remember you're changing a mental habit that has been with you for a lifetime. But habits can be changed.

Summary

We've REVEALED that Scarcity is the number one reason you don't have enough of all the things you want in your life. It's so easy to justify that the reasons are elsewhere, and have nothing to do with you. But they've got everything to do with you and what you perceive as your reality.

How do you obtain the abundance you desire? By understanding the only reason you don't have what you want is because you've been focusing on the wrong things, on what you don't have, and that's where you've put all your energy. As amazing as it is, if you start focusing only on what you have now, gratefully, and what you see yourself having—without one thought that you don't have it yet—you will start to have what you want. This is a universal law, and one that we all need to live by.

Warning: This does not mean you go into debt because you feel sorry for yourself. We have both been guilty of spending because we were depressed—using spending as a drug. In fact, the more depressed you are, the more you may spend and the more you'll be depressed and in debt. Stop the cycle by addressing the low self-worth and lack of vision in your life. Nobody ever spent their way into self-worth—not for very long. Because as soon as you feel good with the new car, house or coat, someone will have one bigger and better and newer. In fact, the first rule of accumulating wealth is to get out of debt. Stop paying all that interest on credit cards, when you could save money and get the bank to pay you interest. If you're broke, in debt and wanting more, you'll have to take an oath of self-control. Stop spending. Start saving. Always share what you can.

Now is the time to start creating abundance. See yourself as someone who has everything in life she needs, and then keep that vision firmly in mind during the day. ACT on that vision by giving where you can: five minutes of your time, a compliment, an old piece of clothing to Salvation Army. When reality tells you otherwise, keep going back to that positive vision. While you're conditioning your mind to see all the opportunities for financial growth, look at two things you can do today to start building financial independence: talk with a financially savvy friend, check out a book from the library, decide not to use your credit card this week, etc. Couple the attitude with the action, and the RESULTS will be you'll be amazed at the abundance/wealth you'll start to bring into your life.

CHAPTER SEVEN
The Monster Lie Satisfaction

The truth Satisfaction doesn't want you to know:
Ask not, have not.

We're going to REVEAL how this Monster beguiles you into believing you have no right to ask. By using guilt and denial, Satisfaction often sabotages your personal and professional successes. So how do you begin, how should you ACT to defeat Satisfaction? We will show you a template you can use to get incredible RESULTS. You'll be able to ask for what you want, starting today!

Meet the Monster Satisfaction

Waiting politely is a good way to get passed by. Is it true that all things come to those who wait? Sure, but only what's left over from those who hustle. We were taught a set of rules and standards, which include the idea that children should be seen and not heard. As grownup "children" we still carry around part of that paradigm telling us we should find ways to get what we want without causing waves.

Not only must we speak out and be bold in order to get what we want and need; it is our right, our inheritance. If you never ask and always wait for others to give to you, there's a very good likelihood you won't get what you want. Being good enough and cute enough and nice enough is not a guarantee for reward. In fact, many times people have noticed they get bypassed because they don't speak out.

The squeaky wheel gets the grease. Tooting your own horn may seem rude, but it is a good way to be heard. We're not saying we condone rude or abrasive behavior. Most of us, when pushed to it, may be able to ask for the needs of others—such as when our children need something. But we aren't even on the list. We seem paralyzed when it comes to taking care of ourselves.

Satisfaction's Voice

Satisfaction reminds you in a shrill little voice of what you were told as a child: it's selfish and bad manners to ask. After all, if you're considerate and wait, you may get what you need. Then again, you may not. Satisfaction believes you must do a lot of wishing and just hope people can read your mind or your body language. In the process, you're deprived of what you need and want, whether it's a second helping of food, a report that's due or help in deciphering information.

What keeps people from asking for what they need? Satisfaction has been giving us some very inaccurate information. Have you ever heard:

It's rude to ask for anything.
Wait until you've been offered.
Don't take seconds, even if you're hungry. It's impolite.
Don't ask a question. They'll know you don't know.
You're not listening if you have to ask that.
You're always asking for something.
Stop bothering people with your needs.

Satisfaction Exercise 1

When did you stop asking for what you needed? Were you told as a child it was impolite to ask if the answer was no? The only way we know to get what we want, is to ask for things. List here things that you feel are impolite to ask for, and then list who told you so.

Example:

Don't ask for: *Seconds on dessert*

Where did I hear that?   *My mother*

Don't ask for:_____

Where did I hear that?_____

Don't ask for:_____

Where did I hear that?_____

Don't ask for:_____

Where did I hear that?_____

Don't ask for:_____

Where did I hear that?_____

Visualizing Satisfaction

Satisfaction is a wimpy, whining Monster that looks like a camel with an ostrich head to keep buried in the sand. Translucent fur allows It to blend into the scenery. Satisfaction is very sure that It should never ask for things and never set boundaries. Satisfaction is sure It never really deserves anything and is positive you should follow Its example.

There is a misconception that if you stick to your guns and ask for what you want, you will be perceived as overly aggressive, selfish and not a team player. If you're lucky, you'll get what you need. Quite the contrary. If you don't ask for what you want you will probably lead a life of quiet desperation, becoming more and more stressed as time goes by.

Asking is healthy, more often than not getting you what you need. Asking helps alleviate the stress because you don't just sit there; you take action and do something. The truth is you can learn to deal with a flat out *no*. You can get past the rejection and see the lesson. You can learn how to handle *no*. There's always a pretty good chance you'll either get a *yes*, or a partial *yes*. You never know until you ask, and it's your right to do so. Everyone in sales knows that selling starts with the word *No*—which often means *not right now*.

How Does Satisfaction Limit You?

There's a big problem in our culture with asking for what we need. Asking is pushy and uncouth; it means we can't do it ourselves, are needy or weak. Asking says we don't have the knowledge and might look foolish if we inquire in the wrong way. Therefore, we have much invested in keeping our mouths shut. Satisfaction plays on this knowledge, knowing it's safer to keep quiet than to have what we want in life. And what a price we pay!

In the beginning, we knew how to ask. As three-year-olds, we were experts in asking. Have you ever witnessed a small child in the cereal aisle at the grocery store?

"Mommy, can I have the Boo-Berry?"

The answer is "No."

Then, without hesitation, the request is reformatted: "Mommy, can I have the Captain Crunch?"

The answer again is "No."

"Fruit Loops?"

"No."

"Sugar Pops?"

"No."

"Cheerios?"

"No."

Now for the finale, a bit of hamming it up: "Frosted Flakes taste *Grrrrr-eat!*" and a sweet, toothy smile. That usually gets a reaction, if not a purchase. Wonder if the volume of sales in certain sweetened cereals is related to how far along the aisle the product is placed?

Three-year-olds are still untouched by social convention. They just keep asking in the face of rejection. In a less forceful way, could you imagine being as persistent? If your car salesman says he can't upgrade the stereo for the same price as the one that comes in the car, think about asking twelve times with more energy, humor and a bigger smile.

Satisfaction Exercise 2

Decide something you really want, i.e. a nicer roommate, a raise, a better car, or to quit hyperventilating when you have to speak in front of people. On a sheet of paper, write that "want" at the top. Then draw a vertical line down the middle. On one side write *Cost* at the top, the other side *Payoff.*

Now list all the ways not having this *Want* is costing you. Having a roommate that you don't want costs you joy and peace of mind, freedom to express yourself, etc. On the other side, write all the ways you're justifying this: the payoff of why you're still tolerating this situation. With the roommate, maybe the payoff means not having to put out energy to find a new person, not having to deal with the unknown (Is the next one worse than this one?), etc. Look at your list and determine when you're willing to begin asking for what you want to change this situation. Now make a pledge to spend five minutes every morning this week looking at alternative ways to handle this problem. There *are* solutions!

If we haven't already been brainwashed enough with Satisfaction, keep in mind it's hard to understand it's okay to ask for everything we want in life and that this isn't selfish. It's our right to speak up and ask. We may be told *no,* but how else will we know? This does not mean we're not wonderful people. There is no right or wrong about asking. We're entitled to get out there and keep on asking in a non-aggressive way. It's a form of selling. You should never apologize for selling. Selling is a conversation about needs and surplus; that's all. Some will label you pushy or rude, but others will call you assertive and ambitious. It's up to you to decide if you really care what people think, because this is when Satisfaction can whisper societal nonsense in your ear that stops you from making smart choices.

Facing the Monster Satisfaction: Our Stories

Sally

As I went down for the second time, I thought, "This is not the way I want to die."
I was in Ft. Lauderdale, Florida and had decided to

try a scuba dive to a shipwreck. I went on a stormy day because it would be a lousy beach day and the fact that there were four-foot waves didn't mean anything to me—yet. I was thinking, heck, I'll be underwater, so what do I care? What I didn't realize is that a boat bouncing around on four-foot waves is apt to bob around a lot. By the time I was suited up, I was already very seasick. My fellow divers included three guys from the circus who were high-wire artists and four guys who were Navy SEALS. This was another warning sign I decided to ignore. These men were so fit you could bounce quarters off their stomachs. I was a five-foot-two, middle-aged lady who usually did thirty-foot dives to watch the pretty fish.

When we went down, it was all I could do to keep these guys in sight. It was deep, dark and cold. I was shivering in my rubber suit and dizzy from nausea. The visibility wasn't more than twelve feet. I remember thinking, "Keep the tips of their flippers in sight at all times." Nobody even noticed whether I was there or not. At last the divemaster signaled it was time to go up. I got up to a place where you're supposed to hover so your blood gases can regulate, about ten feet below the surface. Then, I started to vomit into my regulator, the mouthpiece where your air comes from. I realized I would have to surface. Scenes from a sponge diver movie starring Anthony Quinn filled my mind. There were these Greek divers who came up too suddenly, got covered with ice chips, but died of the bends anyway.

I was losing consciousness and decided to kick up to the surface, bends or not. No easy job since it happens that four-foot waves on the surface mean turbulence at least six feet down.

As I surfaced and gasped for real air, my problems con-

tinued. First of all, the jacket you wear is supposed to inflate like an inner tube with the pull of a tab. That didn't happen. Next, the boat wasn't visible because of the now ten-foot swells. Also, I was getting colder and colder, and hypothermia was setting in. I was numb, violently sick and sinking. I remember getting a mouthful of water and thinking I should scream for help.

Then a curious thing happened. The Committee inside my brain—led by the Monster Satisfaction—decided to hold a meeting to discuss whether this was truly serious enough to ask for help.

In my childhood, I was trained never to clown around in the water and that included never, ever yelling for help unless you were drowning. So, I had a very deep groove in my record that said, "Don't call for help unless you really, really mean it." The people who trained me—parents and relatives—would read the story of "The Little Boy Who Cried Wolf" and suggest that little boys and girls who were foolish enough to cry for unneeded help would be eaten by wolves.

There I was in high waves out at sea, sinking, all the while trying to decide whether I was truly drowning. What if I could make it to the boat after I yelled help? What if I really was all right after all? Then the Committee in my brain suggested that the only way to know if it was a true emergency was to drown. Then I'd know if I should have called for help.

That's when it occurred to me this was no way to die. At the same time a very timid little voice on the Committee spoke up and suggested a near-drowning might count as "significant enough" to allow me to call for help. If I was wrong, I could always live with the humiliation of being a

151

wimp. This all happened in a few quick seconds, but it was like slow motion at the time.

I decided to call for help. I opened my mouth and a squeaky little voice whispered a suggestion for help. Those of you who've heard me speak know I barely need a microphone in a large auditorium, but it was the best I could do from fear of asking wrongly. I tried again, the weight of the scuba tank pulling me down. It was now at least an audible voice. Finally, I was actually able to scream until someone jumped in and pulled me aboard.

Not all asking is so critical, but we need to practice all day long to build up our asking muscles.

Jennifer

"'The free breakfast is only for executive suite members," said the clerk matter-of-factly as she straightened papers and turned to leave.

My daughter Marlo and I were traveling from New York City to Florida, and after driving about nine hours we decided to stop for the night in a little town in South Carolina. Noticing large billboards for several hotels including Holiday Inn, Hampton Inn and Howard Johnson's—all offering free breakfasts—we picked a hotel and went in to register. I asked the clerk what I needed to do to get our free breakfast coupons. That's when we were informed that there was a catch to the free breakfast offer. It was about that time I noticed out of the corner of my eye that my daughter was rapidly distancing herself from me, in anticipation of a rather heated discussion.

I simply asked, in a quiet voice, for the breakfast

coupons, stating that I held this hotel in the highest esteem, and that obviously what they represented here was dishonest advertising, and there must be some mistake. I went on talking, and we ended up getting a wonderful buffet breakfast with do-it-yourself omelets, fruits, juices, and a wide variety of entrees. The best part of all was that it was free, as advertised. All I had to do was ask and stand my ground.

Sally

The rumor in Hollywood circles is that more than once Whoopi Goldberg has bypassed casting directors and called up producers directly asking for parts. Who can forget her Broadway performance in A Funny Thing Happened on the Way to the Forum, *a part usually played by a white male. This tenacity is her hallmark, which is why I wasn't surprised when I saw the following interchange at a book signing for her on Sunset Strip. The lady in front of me pushed a big manila folder at Whoopi and begged, "Please read my film script." Most times I've seen stars take such offerings and toss them, or managers step in and tell these people to back off. Whoopi answered, "The best way to get that considered is to send it to my agent, and put a note that I said to send it."*

She rewarded the tenacity of others. She encouraged this lady not only to ask, but told her where to ask. Go Whoopi!

Satisfaction Exercise 3

One thing we teach in our seminars is an easier way to say *no*. If you know how to say *no,* you may not be so afraid of asking. You can even teach people how to say *no* to you! This works very effectively because you're telling people what you can do, not what you can't. It's a simple three part formula:

I can do _____
(some part that addresses their need that's feasible)

I can't do_____
(what they asked for and why)

And next time_____
(come up with a solution for the future)

Example: Sally: "Hey Jennifer will you loan me fifty dollars?"

Jennifer: "I can show you where the closest ATM machine is. I can't loan you money. I don't loan money to friends. I've found it causes problems. Next time let's talk about budgets before you get into a jam."

Or

Jennifer: "Sally, I need you right now to come and help me carry this."

Sally: "I can come in ten minutes, but I can't right now. I'm finishing up with a client. Next time, if you give me a fifteen minute 'heads up,' then I can arrange my schedule to help you carry those things."

Get the idea? It is a way to keep communication channels open. Five times during the day, try answers using the "I can/can't" formula when you're going to say you cannot do something. You'll be surprised how much easier it seems than just saying "No."

Jennifer

Often, all it takes is asking the same question but to a different person. I can think of more than once when I wanted to use my frequent flier miles for a ticket. When I called the airlines, I was told the dates I requested were blacked out, and couldn't be used. Then I called right back to check on some different dates, got a different person, of course, and this time was told "No problem" in getting tickets for my originally requested dates. Sometimes no doesn't mean no. Remember, there are occasions when no means not right now.

Satisfaction Exercise 4
Ask outrageously.

A friend of ours was earning $1000 for her work, and after taking a course on possibilities, she decided she had everything to gain and nothing to lose by asking an outrageous—to her at the time—amount, because she felt she deserved it and she could handle the *no's*. So she asked for $7000 and got it. This doesn't mean you should charge into your boss's office and demand a fifty percent pay raise, but a reminder that often, not only do we not ask for what we want and deserve, but when we do ask we're meek and ask for less than we can have. Think outrageously for one thing you would like. Decide you can handle the subsequent *yes* or *no* and go for it.

Satisfaction Exercise 5
Understand the impact of *No.*

Often we take it personally, which is why great salespeople

separate the *no* from any personal implications. Their prospect doesn't want to buy the product or service, but they don't see it as a rejection aimed at themselves. Also decide that *no* isn't always *no*. It might mean any number of other things. But the easiest thing to say when asked for something is often the knee-jerk answer, "No." Finally, decide you will not care what people think of you when you ask a specific question. In fact, try this question on five more people. Before you make your request, each time remind yourself you have no vested interest in the answer. You're training your subconscious to focus on a goal regardless of the outcome.

Jennifer

One of the best examples of asking involves something that happened to me in Washington, DC. I got lost, called from my rental car and got directions to the hotel. Seconds later, as I followed the hotel's explicit directions and turned left at a light, I was pulled over by a policeman and given a ticket. When I told him I didn't do anything wrong, he told me I couldn't turn left at the light between 4:00 and 6:00 p.m. I didn't know and couldn't see any sign.

After getting the $50 ticket, I drove to the hotel and told the clerk since I felt they were partially responsible for my ticket due to their directions, would they please pay for my parking for the night? Nope, different owner of the parking concession. Okay, would they consider buying me dinner and breakfast? Yes, they would. I felt somewhat vindicated.

So often we're taught once is too much and to continue asking is boorish, poor manners and certainly not acceptable, but courteously continuing to seek a solution can ultimately pay off.

Cultural training is strong. There's a misleading fairy tale about a little boy who went out one night to play with the fairies in the woods. At the end of the night they gave him a choice: did he want to take the gift they offered—a handful of rocks—or something else, like some diamonds. Naturally, the "greedy" little boy took the diamonds.

Another little boy joined the fairies for games and dancing the next night. Again, at the end of the night, he was offered a fistful of diamonds or a few rocks. He graciously accepted the rocks and went home. When the "greedy" boy awoke, his diamonds had turned to dirty old rocks The gracious little boy found the rocks he chose turned into diamonds.

So the deep, lasting message is that you're a better person and better things will come to you if you take what life hands you and don't reach for more. This is the type of story that brainwashed children so they grew into adults who couldn't or wouldn't ask for what they needed. Polite? Yes, but unsuccessful and unhappy.

Sally

If we know who we are and like who we are, then we believe we have the right to ask. I thought of this when I saw Pearl Bailey in 1967 in the first all-black cast of "Hello Dolly" in Washington, DC. She was born to play Dolly, even if others didn't know it yet. Or, as Ms. Bailey once said:

"There's a period of life when we swallow a knowledge of ourselves and it becomes either good or sour inside."

Satisfaction Exercise 6

Make a list of five things you want more than anything else this year. Now, next to each thing write down five people you can ask for help. Next to the person's name, put their phone number and the date by which you will make contact. Note: we did not say a date by which you will just call them. Anyone can leave a message on a machine. We're talking about real, one-on-one contact that allows you the time to make a request.

What You Want:_____

Name/Number:_____ By When :_____

What You Want:_____

Name/Number:_____ By When :_____

What You Want:_____

Name/Number:_____ By When :_____

What You Want:_____

Name/Number:_____ By When :_____

What You Want:_____

Name/Number:_____ By When :_____

Fill this in now! Make the first request within twenty-four hours. There are tricks to teach your mind how to be smarter and work more quickly when it comes to asking. The first step is to know that asking is not rude—that you deserve good things and that people also have a right to say *no*.

Asking is an accelerated approach to having all that you want. Asking is the quickest way to be successful, yet many people don't get it. Instead, they seem to think the way to be smart is to look as if you know it all and have it all. That is the height of stupidity, but it is a strong message we get from society.

Satisfaction Exercise 7
Create an "asking" well.

Wishing wells are for fools and lovers. Folks throw in a coin and hope for the best. So who is going to put things in order for this to come true—the goldfish at the bottom?

But what if you stack the deck? Start by listing everything you want on slips of paper, and put them in a symbolic well: a hat box, salad spinner or whatever you like. Pull out one of the items and decide what five places you could start asking for this particular thing. Maybe you want a pair of genuine cowboy boots. Well, you could call the manufacturer. Call a Western store and ask about sales. Call a thrift store. Hang around a cowboy bar or a stable. Or you could read the obituaries. You could put up an ad in the grocery store. You could offer a swap: will baby-sit for boots; will weed for boots. You could stop everybody you see with boots and tell them you like their boots and you would like a pair, can they help you?

Satisfaction Exercise 8

Get your right brain into gear by creating a "can have" collage. The point here is that we often get so used to denying our dreams and suppressing even the mildest desire, all in the name of reality. We've totally conditioned ourselves not to think big, not to dream, not to be aware of what we want and are entitled to. So begin by ripping pictures from magazines of things you'd like to do or have. Perhaps you've dreamed of canoeing but believe it's too expensive, too dangerous or you don't have anyone who'll go with you and don't know who to ask. Maybe you'd like a briefcase, college education, new tennis racquet. Paste what you'd like onto a big poster and hang it where you can see it every day. This visualization can turn dreams and goals into reality. It works because you begin training your brain to select things you might have missed.

Satisfaction Exercise 9

Ask yourself "What if?" As we get used to asking, we expand our right brain by asking "What if" questions. What if dogs kept people on leashes? What if clocks ran backwards? What if all jewelry was edible—you get the picture. We can overcome the Monster Satisfaction's ugly little reminders not just by questioning, but through *outrageous* questions that will open up new ideas.

Think of ten absurd "What ifs." Then look at a present challenge and use the "What if" exercise. What if somebody wanted to swap boating lessons for cooking lessons? Sally has swapped cooking lessons for a house-share in the Hamptons, swimming lessons for Spanish lessons and yardwork for recording studio time.

List what you want. Decide who has that to offer. Then figure out what you have that you can barter.

Satisfaction Exercise 10

Try the "worst first" approach. What's the worst answer you can get when you ask? The worst thing you can think of that could happen? Can you take it? If so, you've set yourself up for success already. Write down four answers that would be awful to hear, followed by your responses.

Answer:_____

Response:_____

Answer:_____

Response:_____

Answer:_____

Response:_____

Answer:_____

Response:_____

Reminders

A Two-Way Street.

We give and give, and then we feel it's okay to ask. Mind you, we must give for the sake of giving, but it teaches our subconscious that giving is half of a two-way street. The best way to get when you ask is to build a loop of cooperation.

Even the Bible says: "Ask and it shall be given you; seek and ye shall find; knock, and it shall be opened unto you." Matthew 7:7.

Your Action Plan

Remember, if we buy into what others believe we should do, we'll still be waiting for permission to have what we want when they're putting flowers on our graves. Determine you'll begin right now asking for and getting what you want, despite what anyone else thinks.

When asking for help try three things:

✓ After you say hello, cut the small talk and tell them you're calling to ask something of them. This forces you to ask instead of getting nervous and saying nothing. Also, they won't feel cheated that you were chatting them up and suddenly—Wham!—you really called because you wanted something. You can always visit later.

✓ Explain in two or fewer sentences what you want. You can even write this out as a script and read it.

✓ Tell the person on the other end that you want them to feel free to say yes or no, but if they say no, would they be willing to suggest two other people you could ask? Let your right brain do the work. Visualize what you want.

Summary

We've REVEALED that you've been trapped by the belief

that asking is not good. When you buy into this Satisfaction assumption, it's a virtual guarantee you won't be as successful, happy or productive as you'd like. Now imagine someone offers you a key, and every time you need anything—a question answered, a seat on a bus, a favor, a raise—you use your key to unlock all the possibilities simply by asking. When you understand this, and start asking on a daily basis, you'll immediately start to see positive changes.

ACT now! Look at three specific areas in which you can begin to ask: talking to a manager about leaving on time instead of being forced to work late; clarification on a bill; requesting a different glass of wine/juice/milk because the one you have doesn't taste right to you. Start small to look after your needs. Without asking you can pretty much guarantee you won't get what you want, and when you begin to ask, to look out after yourself as the unique, independent woman who deserves to have whatever she's asking for, you'll start to see RESULTS, usually much sooner than you imagine.

CHAPTER EIGHT

The Monster Lie Experteaser

The truth Experteaser doesn't want you to know:
*Experts know a lot about things in the past, but nobody
has lived the future yet!*

W e're going to REVEAL how this Monster tricks you into denying your intuition, your body, your instinct—often putting you in great jeopardy personally and professionally. We'll show you how to ACT immediately to trust your own expertise. The RESULTS of trusting yourself include: seeking the right information, getting the right support, and regaining the control you never knew you'd given away.

Meet the Monster Experteaser

No quality is more essential to growth than hope, nothing more devastating than the removal of that hope. Take away someone's hope in the hospital, and that's the person likely to suffer a relapse. Take away a person's hope in any situation, and her morale suffers greatly, she loses interest, becomes lethargic, quits trying, and often suffers illness or physical symptoms as manifestations of stress.

Experteaser's Voice

Experteaser is a know-it-all who warns you that you'd

better put all your trust in the experts. It's that nagging little voice that encourages you to trust blindly the old proven way of doing things: always check with everyone else and never go with your gut instinct. Experteaser preaches that doctors, managers, scientists, ministers and anyone older or younger or with more knowledge knows more than you, and can probably do things more efficiently or better than you. If you want to know whether you have your very own Experteaser, see if any of these statements sound familiar:

We've always done it this way.
Don't fix what's not broken.
You can't fight City Hall.
I've forgotten more than you'll ever learn.
Listen first; eventually you'll be qualified to respond.
How could you know more than an expert?
You're just a beginner!
Don't question years of experience.
Don't try that or you'll be disappointed.

Experteaser Exercise 1

Which expert has kept you from spreading your wings? List here some of the things experts told you that kept you from exploring or going forward:

1. _____

2. _____

3. _____

4. _____

---

5. _____

6. _____

7. _____

8. _____

9. _____

10. _____

Visualizing Experteaser

Experteaser appears as a large, important-looking laboratory rat, standing up on Its two back legs. It has a worldly and knowledgeable air. Of course, It's just one of many rodents pushing through the maze of life. Just because Experteaser got through one maze doesn't mean It can get you through yours. What's painfully clear about experts, upon close examination, is that they are often only experts on the past.

You can also see shades of Experteaser in your professor, brother, favorite movie star or family member. It sounds important and pompous, but the really important thing here is It can be wrong—even if It has six college degrees or has written twenty-six books. Experteaser wants you to believe It knows what's best for you. Don't swallow Its Lie. Few experts have power over the future. In this day and age, information is moving so rapidly, an expert may only have valuable insight for a few months.

How Does Experteaser Limit You?

No one likes to reinvent the wheel. Most people will take

the advice or follow the path of an expert because it seems less stressful. Why invent a better mousetrap? The old ones are fine, until we get infested with mice and need a new approach. Human nature usually tells us to accept the current way of doing things. Why expend extra energy? Why forge a new path, especially if we have to put our reputations on the line in the process?

We are a nation that believes in experts. This societal conditioning is prevalent in everything we do. Every television news show brings in experts to tell us how to cope or handle situations. Most businesses bring in the guru of the moment. Many commercials rely on experts to tell us what we should take to feel healthy. In the process we've denied our own common sense or logic.

Experteaser Exercise 2

Think of all of the people who had to relearn skills. Typewriter experts, architectural artists, illustrators, engravers are now learning requisite computer skills. To remind yourself how quickly the world changes—and how experts come and go—list five things that are obsolete or no longer used: Example: Milkman deliveries, eight-track cassettes, Beta video format.

1. _____

2. _____

3. _____

4. _____

5. _____

Should you seek out those with knowledge? You bet! Should you assume their word is law? Never! You must listen as if their information is a part of the combination to the solution, not necessarily *the* solution. If your problem is a combination lock, you need more than one number to open it, you need a set of numbers, a combination (of information) to get what you need. It's vital not to assume someone with authority in a certain area can or should tell you how to run your life.

Christy is an award-winning photographer who went from obscurity to recognition—not to mention an income increase—when she finally ditched the expert who tried to undo her. She was in photography school, and her professor was to review her work. The professor started the review session by announcing with certainty that Christy should get out of photography altogether. She had no talent and was wasting her time. Because she was an older student in her mid-thirties, she had the presence of mind to inform the professor she disagreed with his analysis. Christy went on to photograph the great National Parks of the Southwest for her award-winning work—but only after she went home and cried for an entire summer, doubting her talent. Through the support of family and friends she tried her skills anyway. Boy, was that expert wrong. It ought to be against the law to discourage people with a dream. By the way, the professor gave up teaching and went into administration work.

Facing the Monster Experteaser: Our Stories

Jennifer

"Your son has slight brain damage."
When my son, Michael, was in his early teens, he had

learning problems, including dyslexia. We took him to a well-known neurologist in order to get a diagnosis of any physical problems that might be interfering with his ability to learn.

That was the evening I learned that my son had minor brain damage. The doctor suspected it was due to a very high fever Michael had experienced as a baby. He called me into his office and told me in a very authoritative voice—at least that's the way it sounded to me—that my son should not expect to go to college; that a nice vocational school was really the best we could hope for.

I went out of his office in shock, but pretty soon my brain kicked in, and I asked myself—why should my son settle for a nice vocational school? College seemed a better option for him. So, I conveniently forgot to tell him what the doctor had said. Lucky for me, because Michael went on to graduate school and completed his work in Forensic Science. Yes, he received his Masters Degree—and with a 4.0 grade point average to boot!

Don't listen to the experts without checking out their credentials; without confirming your heart! You will be told how to live, what stocks to buy, what your child should or shouldn't do, what operations to have and not have and what oil to put in your car.

Sally

My favorite expert story is of my own business. I was told by at least three experts in public speaking that I could not start a business with less than $100,000 in the bank and $20,000 in promotional materials.

> *I started my business on $20 worth of business cards and three stapled ink jet printed pages describing my work. If you include my fax and phone, I spent about $500 the first year. Within that year, I billed $60,000. The next year I bought a computer for $3,000. If you add about another $1000 in expenses—phone bills, stamps, etc.—I spent $4000 to bring in three international clients, which brought my billings to six figures.*

It's gotten to the point that if experts tell the two of us something is a bad idea, we rush out and do it. Experts get left in the dust when technology or conditions change. It's not that knowledge and experience don't count, it's just that our culture has had a way of making deities out of experts. We love to follow someone else who is doing the thinking for us. We like to cut corners. Hear what the experts have to say, then weigh the information before going forward.

Experteaser Exercise 3

List five things that you need. Eliminate "want" because we're working on programming the mind to believe these are obtainable.

1. Begin with one of your five goals and list below:
   Example: *money for college tuition, for car repairs, rent money, a publisher, a job.*

   _____

2. Visualize a wagon wheel with spokes all around the hub and draw it on a piece of paper.
3. Write your goal in the center, along with a picture. Stick figures are fine.

---

4. Each day for a week, add five additional pictures or thoughts on how to get this and who you can ask. These are the spokes of the wheel.

5. At the end of two days you will have many different ideas and approaches to stimulate your right brain into action.

Exercise tips:

☞ Use words and pictures together

☞ Use different colored markers

☞ Keep this "chart" on the wall in plain view, in order to stimulate yourself to action. This is also a good methodology for office teams to use in brainstorming.

☞ Understand how powerful this is in allowing the brain to make its own connections and come up with combinations you never even dreamed of.

Why should we challenge experts? The reason is that frequently they're wrong. Not only is their expertise often *passé*; they can't predict our success or failures. They can only make educated guesses as to the outcome of a certain venture.

Nowhere is this truer than in the American University system. There are so many horror stories we thought of creating a special punishment—perhaps special jails—for teachers who demoralize young people who have dreams. How dare teachers tell young people they have no talent? Some of the greatest artists, singers and athletes of our day were slow starters.

Experts are only people who are supposedly knowledgeable in certain areas. That doesn't give them the right to play God, so for pity sakes, don't elevate them above their accomplishments. Even experts aren't able to score one hundred percent their whole life.

Every time you hear someone say the following, it's a big clue there's room in your field for some innovative ideas:

That's not your department.
We tried it and it doesn't work.
That's not what we do here.
Who do you think you are?
It's impossible. No one has ever done that.

Remember, the people on the inside of an organization have made their money or acquired fame doing things a certain way. Change means they might not be on top anymore. Where is the incentive to give your new ideas a try? It is an expensive risk. They are comfortable, and they probably have no altruistic need to share the goods at the top with you.

Jennifer

Be aware that Experteaser does not go away when we get older and wiser and feel as if we should know better. One example is my belief in my inability to speak French. Now let me explain how this mentality can linger and affect so many things we do. For years I studied French; two years at the Alliance Francaise in New York, one of the best French schools in the country. I took a year of private classes as well as some French in high school and college.

But in my French class, I prefaced all my conversations with, "I know I'm not very good . . . ." One day, one of my fellow students turned to me and said angrily, "Jennifer, will you stop it. Not only are you constantly putting down your ability to speak, but you're affecting everyone else in class!" Finally, I let go of the voice telling me I couldn't be any good so I'd better knock myself before anyone else did.

When I finally let go of this belief, I could speak the language—not necessarily with great aplomb, but I was able to make myself understood when my daughter and I were in Paris. It was with great joy I realized the only reason I hadn't been able to speak French was because I convinced myself I couldn't.

Sally

I remember the day my friend Joyce called to tell me her husband had started a game company. Steve and his friends had decided to create a game called Star Crossed, a trivia game about movies, Hollywood and celebrities. If you're a movie buff, this is your game. Steve and his partners decided there were a lot of movie buffs, especially given the home video business. They were right. Their game was one of the hottest selling games in 1996. But that was after people told them they couldn't break into the game business and go against the likes of Milton Bradley and Parker Brothers. In fact, that's the way they first tried to go with their game idea and were told to leave the product in the protective care of big corporate America.

Instead, they took their product and did all their own production and marketing. It's a wonderful game, but, better yet, is the bigger game they won, called, "Let's blow off the experts and create some history." Their product launch was at none other than FAO Schwartz toy store in New York City.

173

How do you outthink the experts—and never even have to go back to school? We need tricks to shake up our brain cells. Some research says we use only four percent of our brain—yes, that's the latest statistic—leaving a whopping ninety-six percent on tap.

Jennifer

I demonstrate this in my seminars by asking two people to come up with a combination number, and in less than three seconds, I give the audience fifteen combinations that add up to their number. It's pretty impressive. I do it to remind everyone how many combinations/ways we've got to go after and get what we want.

Women have always been breaking rules and debunking myths. In her book *Uppity Women of the Renaissance,* Vicki Leon tells the story of Miss Celia Fiennes, a women who dabbled at being a lady-in-waiting but was bored out of her gourd. So, she went on expeditions to coal mines, caves and archeological sites, survived falls with her horse, eluded road bandits, and in 1697, completed her longest journey—six hundred miles in six weeks.

Experteaser Exercise 4

In order to create a change in any area, start with an idea of something you'd like to accomplish. Then ask yourself:

☞ How long could that take? (List in hours or days or weekends.)

☞ How much money will that take?

☞ Who is waiting for this innovation?

☞ Who will buy this?

☞ How much will they pay for it?

☞ How much will each one/service hour/installation/show cost?

☞ Who else wants to see it happen? Do they have money?

☞ How else can I get backing: foundations, partnerships, loans?

☞ What stopped other people from doing this?

☞ And most importantly . . . what would stop me?

Right now, choose one thing that you're determined to change in your life. Then schedule ten minutes every day—no exceptions—for the next two weeks and work on it.

At the end of that time, evaluate what you've done and decide how you're going to proceed. While you're performing this exercise, any time you hear those "expert voices" getting in your way, just say, "Stop" and shut them out. Everything we accomplish comes in small pieces, small steps, little beginnings. The secret is "keeping on" tomorrow and the day after that. That's how you'll overcome and prove Experteaser wrong, because you'll start seeing results. This enables you to start slowly changing your beliefs. The power that comes from these results is nothing short of miraculous!

Experteaser Exercise 5

There are many, many examples of individuals who chose not to listen to the experts.

Elizabeth Blackwell, the first woman in America to receive a medical degree, was regarded as immoral—or simply mad—by many when she decided she wanted to study medicine. Turned down by Philadelphia and New York City schools, she wrote to a number of small northern colleges, and in 1847, was admitted to the Geneva, New York, Medical College. Her graduation in 1849 was highly publicized.

Florence Nightingale, the founder of modern nursing, came up against tremendous resistance when she decided to go into nursing. At the time, she decided she wanted to work in hospitals instead of embarking on a more privileged life, befitting her social standing. Her family was enraged and tried to stop her from doing what they considered work never done by "ladies," but often women of questionable character. However, because of her persistence, she managed to do some private nursing, and spend time at a German school and hospital. Consequently, in 1853, she became superintendent of the London Institution for Sick Gentlewomen in Distressed Circumstances, which allowed her to achieve independence from her family. She, of course, went on to change the face of nursing.

Write down two things "experts" have told *you* that stopped you from going forward in some way. Now rewrite how the scenario should have ended. Whether you can do anything to change that piece of history or not, look how these voices stop us from moving forward.

Example:

Expert No. 1 said: *"You can't learn Russian."*

If it could be changed: *Could listen to tapes or take class*

Expert No. 1 said: _____

If it could be changed: _____

Expert No. 2 said: _____

If it could be changed: _____

Jennifer

Having my photograph taken with celebrities is usually not my thing, but when I found myself at an event with Margaret Thatcher, and attending a small cocktail party in her honor, I was delighted to be photographed with her. Getting into Parliament at the tender age of thirty-four, Ms. Thatcher was already settled into the "statutory woman's" place in the Cabinet as Education Minister. That wasn't enough for her, however, and in 1975 she challenged Edward Heath for the Tory leadership. When she went into his office to tell him her decision to run, he didn't even look up, but simply said, "You'll lose. Good day to you." The rest is history. She became Britain's first female Prime Minister in 1979.

Experteaser Exercise 6
Believe your own press.

Some of the most successful people on earth are also some of the most surprised. But they know what the Wizard of Oz knew: it's all in the perception. If you give the world an outer show of achievement, you very often can achieve it. It's as if your faith and enthusiasm can create reality. Without a vision, the people perish, so keep your vision alive and well.

And why not? Pessimism has been winning for years by creating failures and by disheartening people. Experts are no more than people who have something to show for their effort. Potential experts are people who're still waiting for the evidence to show up. People who're successful are the ones who can wait the longest for the evidence, while they're acting successful ahead of time.

Right now, start planning your future based on your dream coming true. That means start looking at places to spend or invest your money. Start researching the charities to which you'll give your money, the office where you'll be working, the stateroom where your vacation will begin. Remember to think like someone with a success on their hands.

Now write a newspaper piece on yourself to appear ten years from now. Explain how you accomplished your goal, mention all the people you want to thank for their help, tell what happened along the way and then draw a picture of yourself accepting the appropriate honors.

Jennifer

Faith Popcorn made a name for herself, literally. She created a new name and a new line of business: predicting market trends. I heard her speak often in the late 70s and early 80s at the Sales Executives Club of New York. I watched her courage and vision in inventing and creating herself, and a need for her services. These skills later catapulted her into a highly successful woman in an area predominantly male.

Experteaser Exercise 7
Station Break.

Make up a thirty-second TV commercial and radio spot for your innovations. Decide how you'll go public. Draw it in pictures or storyboards and then use a home video to shoot the boards with you and your friends doing the voices of each part. The more you can simplify your explanation to the public, the clearer your vision will be to you. You could even use the commercial to attract potential investors, whether it's a dog walking service or a new home-based business worth hundreds of thousands of dollars.

Jennifer

Courage is something all of us admire. As a runner, one of the women I admire greatly is Roberta Gibb, who, at twenty-three years old became the first woman to run the Boston Marathon in 1966. However, it wasn't quite as easy as that. No woman was welcome in the Boston

Marathon. In fact, when she requested a race application from the Boston Athletic Association—which governs the Boston Marathon—they unequivocally refused to send her one.

She loved running and decided to enter the race anyway. She rode a Greyhound bus all the way from San Diego to Boston—a three-and-a-half-day trip. All she had to eat the whole time were a few apples. She got to her parents' home in Winchester, Massachusetts the day before, did a little running to stretch, and the next day showed up for the race wearing a hooded sweatshirt to cover her long blonde hair.

Gibb was a runner. The previous summer she ran forty miles in a single day. In 1964, while a student at Wellesley College, she went to watch the Boston Marathon and felt drawn to the runners in an irrational way— much like falling in love, she later reported in an article in Runners' World Magazine.

In order to avoid a confrontation at the starting line, she hid in the woods and joined in as soon as the first runners passed. Then she began to run. She said she believed she conveyed such a sense of joy that nobody hassled her that day. Gibb finished 3.21.40. She said later she could have run a lot faster than she did.

Incidentally, the Boston Athletic Association said it was impossible for a woman to run that far. It would destroy her, or at the very least ruin her chances for having children. That was an established fact, recognized. How wonderful Roberta Gibb—the mother of a son—decided not to listen, and opened the door for women runners around the world.

Experteaser Exercise 8
Genius at work. Do not disturb.

List at least ten great ideas you've had over the years. Now list why you haven't moved forward with each. Did it have anything to do with the "experts" who told you these ideas wouldn't work?

Great Idea: _____

Why I didn't Do It: _____

Great Idea: _____

Why I didn't Do It: _____

Great Idea: _____

Why I didn't Do It: _____

Great Idea: _____

Why I didn't Do It: _____

Great Idea: _____

Why I didn't Do It: _____

Great Idea: _____

Why I didn't Do It: _____

Great Idea: _____

Why I didn't Do It: _____

Great Idea: _____

Why I didn't Do It: _____

Great Idea: _____

Why I didn't Do It: _____

Great Idea: _____

Why I didn't Do It: _____

Experteaser Exercise 9

Interview an expert. Look at someone who seems to have survived and thrived despite the odds. Talk with them. Find out how they handled adversity, how they turned deaf ears to all the advice.

Experteaser Exercise 10

Get a mentor. Call everyone you respect—or write them, or both—until you find someone—it might even be someone you've never met—who will help guide you along as you create change in your life. Note: this is not an expert who will tell you what to do, but someone whose guidance you trust. Someone who's been there before. Find someone who can coach you and shorten your learning curve. Don't stop until you get someone!

Mentor's name: _____

Reminders

Baby Steps.

Many ideas can be created on the installment plan. If you have an idea, see if you can develop a smaller model of it to show potential partners what you have in mind. A prototype, a videotape, a drawing of your ideas, all of these will help you bring your dream closer to reality.

Experts don't necessarily know; they're simply people with more knowledge/experience than you have in a certain area. With some exceptions you, too, could become an expert in their field if you begin now reading a book a week on any given subject and continue for ten years. Learn from experts but do not genuflect at their office doors.

Inspiration.

It's been said, genius is ten percent inspiration and ninety percent perspiration. It's your energy and tenacity, not intelligence, which divides you from the pack. When experts tell you that you will fail, remember they have no idea how much drive you have. Negative comments from experts show they have no respect for peoples' vulnerability. They either forget what it feels like, or are jealous of people who are daring to go against the grain. If your idea is not right or the timing is wrong, the world will let you know. Then you can adjust your approach.

Keep trying: there is always room for another expert. Countless gifts have been lost to the world in the name of pompous assumption, arrogance and being right, all doled out by the expert who is in a position to help, but has instead hurt and hindered.

Your Action Plan

List the steps it will take to launch at least one of your ideas. Set a date on your calendar to mark when you will take the first five steps. Make step one now. Begin today.

Steps: *Date completed:*

1._____

2._____

3._____

As you are creating your plan ask yourself:

☞ Who has said this idea won't work?

☞ Is this person an expert in exactly the same area?

☞ Can this person predict the future?

☞ Who else do I respect whom I can consult on this idea?

☞ How long am I willing for this to take?

☞ What shortcuts can I take without compromising the quality or outcome?

Summary

We've **REVEALED** how the "experts" have been telling you—for as long as you would listen—that their way is right. This dialogue is responsible for many of the doubts that stop you from succeeding. But the great news is: you can change your future immediately by ACTING as your own adviser, your own parent, the voice that tells you your own instincts and ideas are great, so follow them. This will feel a little—or a lot—strange at first. After all, it's a new habit you're forming. But it's a habit you'll continue to nurture for the rest of your life, because it's a habit that will get you RESULTS.

CHAPTER NINE
The Monster Lie Yardstick

The truth Yardstick doesn't want you to know:
*If you squeeze a square peg into a round hole, it's bound
to get stuck.*

Now let us REVEAL the Monster named Yardstick. It wants you believe you can never measure up to the important standards of the world. Yardstick wants you to think that no matter how hard you try, no matter what you achieve, you'll always fall short. It's time to ACT now. If you learn to control Yardstick, you can get the RESULTS you want. You can achieve even more than ever because you won't be using up precious time trying to please people and their silly notions of what is important.

Meet the Monster Yardstick

Have you ever been to the movies and seen a great comedy and laughed so loud and so hard that others asked you to be quiet? Don't you dare be quiet! You paid good money to enjoy the comedy, and that means laughing out loud. A funny movie is a pretty appropriate place to laugh freely. But some people have a certain picture of just how much laughter is acceptable in a public place. Those people most likely edit every emotion they have so they always live life at half-volume.

Everyone seems to want conformity, and they all want you to conform to them. Stand straight, cut your hair, grow your hair, lower your hem, raise your hem, and on and on they go.

When you start editing your self-expression you're killing your self-esteem; you're killing the essence of yourself, piece by piece. We're not talking about being obnoxious to get attention, but if you want to whistle while you walk, or yodel on the ski slope, or skip on the beach, why not? Who cares what anyone else thinks? Acting cool and sophisticated can get boring. In the movie *Living Outloud*, Holly Hunter's character says to her ex-husband, "I left me before you did."Trying to fit into someone else's picture of "acceptable" will kill off your energy and enthusiasm. It is just that energy you need to make your life happen.

Yardstick's Voice

If you don't allow yourself to bask in goodness in the best of times, how will you ever get through the rest of times? How often do you censor yourself, or listen to others who'd like to tell you how to behave? Listen to Yardstick's sing-song voice, always going up and down to fit the rule of the moment, and see if these sound familiar:

You should have two kids by now.
Why throw your life away on a dead-end job just because
    you like it.
You can't drive a junk car and look successful.
People will judge you by your clothes.
You're too fat.
You must have a college degree.
Don't show your feelings. Don't let 'em see you sweat.

Looking good is important.
Give in to peer pressure. It's just this once.

Yardstick Exercise 1

What words of condemnation about your spirit have you been listening to? Who told you not to giggle, skip, jump, and laugh out loud? How old were you when the editing on your heart, soul and emotions began? List all the ways you've been asked to put a lid on your joy:

Example: *Don't hum while you do that; it's childish.*

1._____

2._____

3._____

4._____

5._____

Visualizing Yardstick

What does Yardstick look like? It's a tall bird with a long, skinny body colored from neck to knee with black inch markings on yellow fur. Yardstick stands up ruler-straight, trying to appear dignified and authoritative. It carries around a big rule book.

How Does Yardstick Limit You?

There are no points in Heaven for stifling your emotions for appearances' sake. Yardstick wants you to think you'll have points taken off for appearing foolish or childlike. Yardstick uses the fear of being humiliated and looking foolish as a club to beat us into conformity. Don't let It!

We're not giving rage-a-holics permission for verbal violence. We're simply saying you may only pass this way once, so why not experience the richness of your life?

Feel the joy of pride, the silliness of a joke, the fun of a windy day. Make a snow angel, cover your feet with sand, wear a silly mask at Halloween and bask in the joy of life. If you let Monster Yardstick have Its way, you'll spend every waking hour trying to look good for others, trying to lose weight or purge, or agreeing with others, and never feeling good about the gift that you are to the world.

Truly following your passions—despite what Yardstick says—is living your life to the highest level. Consider this: What are you saving that life for? Tomorrow? Think again. There are many, many tomorrows that never come. If we silence the Yardstick Monster, we've got a glorious day today.

Yardstick Exercise 2

List five occupations you think you could enjoy, that wouldn't even feel like work:

Example: Rock star.

1. _____

2. _____

3. _____

4. _____

5. _____

There may be a piece of these occupations that you *can* do, or a combination of all of them.

One other note here. Yardstick, as we well know, doesn't just speak through those around us. Our own inner voices get in our way as much or more than those of others. Have you ever hit a lousy shot in tennis and told yourself you're an imbecile, that you know you have to keep your eye on the ball, follow through, get there early, etc.? Have you ever said the wrong thing to a boss and told yourself you might as well start sprucing up your résumé again if you keep up those stupid remarks? Often, this is not our true dialogue, but a collection of voices we've accumulated over the years— teachers, authority figures, bosses and others who "knew" what was in our own best interest and lost no time in telling us so.

Yardstick wants you to live up to others' expectations and by all means don't think that you can judge what's right for your life. No, choosing your life's goals is way too important to be left up to *you.* So Lies Yardstick.

It says you should consult your wise uncle, magazines, TV sitcoms, teachers, gurus and the stars (psychics) to know what is the perfect plan for your life.

"Watch out,"Yardstick says. "Don't ask yourself what makes you happy, or else the next thing you know, you'll be saying what's on your mind, disagreeing with your mother-in-law's unkind remark, ordering the food you like—messy though it is—and doing as you please with no thought to pro- tocol. Okay. You'll be happy, but will you look good? Isn't that all Yardstick cares about?

You could spend endless anxious hours performing mind- less tasks because it pleases everyone to do things the way they've always been done. This will keep you so busy you'll have no energy to invent new and better ways to produce results for yourself and your loved ones. In this way you can measure up to others' expectations and never be happy. If you believe Yardstick, you'll spend a great deal of energy trying to measure up to other people's expectations—which, by the way, they can rarely measure up to themselves.

Facing the Monster Yardstick: Our Stories

Jennifer

A friend of mine has been stressed out ever since she graduated from college. Judging by the many young people I talk with around the country, she's definitely not the exception. Her parents expected her to continue with the predetermined, focused path that led her to a degree. What they don't understand is that she had the focus to get that degree, but doesn't yet know what she wants to do with her life. She is really struggling—looking, asking, but most of all, feeling like a failure. Yardstick has done a great job here.

All this because she's allowed many people to remind her she's still living with her parents, doesn't have a job yet, and hears "what a pity that her education is going to waste."

Now again, neither Sally nor I are saying to go paddle a canoe all day and eat sunflower raisin cookies, telling everyone that water is your passion and you want to enjoy your life. Unless your passion really is canoeing. In that case, you could find about a hundred ways to earn a living, including: teaching canoeing, writing a book on canoeing for the physically handicapped, turning it into a new exercise and marketing it on talk shows, and on and on. With the cookies you're on your own—unless you have a recipe to sell to Debbi Fields.

Sally

I remember a church leader informing me that real Christians gave ten percent of their income before taxes and didn't need life insurance or fire insurance. I asked if that is how he ran his household. He had to admit he was a couple of prayers short of full faith, and his luxury home was well protected by the Rock. Not Jesus—the Rock of Gibraltar. Why are people so quick to tell others how to live their lives?

Yardstick Exercise 3

List five times you didn't do something the proper way, and what happened?

Example: *Ate the frosting off a cupcake first. World did not end.*

1. _____

2. _____

3. _____

4. _____

5. _____

We're so afraid of letting go because we might be wrong. The problem is, we might miss our lives in the process.

Jennifer

If you grew up believing "Father knows best,"then whatever he said was always right. So when he said you should go to school and be a lawyer, because that's a respectable, lucrative and a prestigious way to earn a living— even if it's not what you wanted to do—you went. No matter that you found law hideously boring, your father said it was the right thing to do.

I remember when it wasn't acceptable for girls to wear slacks to school. Yes, it was more important to look good than keep warm, avoid frostbite or catch cold. It got cold growing up in Missouri in the winter What about office environments where women are forbidden to wear slacks because it isn't professional enough? Yes, they still exist, and these grown-up women who need jobs will also endure snow, ice and discomfort because it's the dress code, the "professional" way to dress.

Society dictates, and so often we jump to attention without questioning. Why, for instance, do so many women still wear high heels? Often, we see women wearing those three-inch numbers to go to corporate events, when in reality they suffer foot pain, back pain, calluses and other afflictions.

Sally

I've always felt a little awkward about dressing up for business. When I wear high heels I feel like a five-year-old playing dress up. I'm never sure I have that pulled-together look I see in my colleagues. I work very hard to achieve the corporate look, including matching earrings, handbag, shoes. But some days you just can't win.

SALLY FRANZ & JENNIFER WEBB

I remember one day in particular when I got a good les-son about Yardstick. I had two interviews that day, one with an ad agency and one with a private Garden Club Foundation. I wore a dark-blue, heavy cotton twill suit with tiny white dots—like a dotted Swiss pattern—and white linen cuffs and collar. It was fashionably short and had great lines. I accented the white trim with pearl jewelry.

After my first interview, the woman from the advertis-ing company said she was glad to hire me for consulting work, but said I needed to do something about my staid schoolteacher wardrobe. In fact, she recommended that I try dressing much more hip. The second interview from the foun-dation said that they were considering me, but were shocked that I wore such a skimpy, immodest, trendy suit to the in-terview.

Same suit, two contrasting Yardsticks. "Hey," I thought, "you people need to get a life!"

Jennifer

I remember attending a symphony once and getting so carried away with the beauty of the music that when one movement ended I burst into applause. Or should I say I burst into applaud. No one else applauded. It wasn't the "correct" time, and so I felt extremely foolish. I hadn't gone along with what was acceptable behavior, I had just got caught up in the moment and expressed my appreciation at the wonderful music.

The message here is very simple: Live to meet others' ex-pectations and your life won't be your own any longer. It will belong to your co-workers, your in-laws, your spouse, signif-icant other, children, boss, mother, best friend, or society at large.

Keep a muzzle on Yardstick and you'll have the freedom you deserve to live life the way you want to live it. Don't forget to live it for today. Don't spend one more second thinking you'll really start "living" as soon as: you're older, retire, finish school, get past this year, etc.

Sally

"Mayday, Mayday!" shouted the captain. "We're going down."

I'd never been on a sinking ship before, but it occurred to me that the biggest problem is to know when to jump off. Deep, cold water isn't much of a choice.

My good friend Marion, a terrific woman, held fundraising parties every summer on an island just off the shoreline of Westport, Connecticut. The parties became legendary. One year we added to the folklore by renting a party boat to Shelter Island, and the boat sank.

We were on this flat party boat when the captain suggested we all stand in the back so we could go faster, letting the bow skim above the water. Halfway across the harbor there was a log floating in the water. The quick-thinking captain slowed the boat down to avoid puncturing the pontoons. However, he forgot to tell us to redistribute our weight.

As we all stood in the back end of our pontooned vessel, water started gushing around our feet like a fire hydrant in the inner city in July. There was much shouting, and we all put on life vests and started to redistribute the weight of our now half-submerged deck. We hailed a nearby boat to come and take passengers to shore. With gusto and bravado, a very tall stockbroker announced, "Women and children first."

I turned to him and asked, "Can you swim?"
He said, "No."

I told him I could swim three miles without a life vest and that shore was only a half-mile. So I simply countered his Hollywood-scripted command by shouting, "Non-swimmers first." This made all the non-swimmers—who were showing definite signs of panic—very happy.

The Yardstick/macho expectation of "women and children first" could have actually cost someone's life. As it turned out, within two hours we were all safe and sound on the island dancing, eating lobsters and greatly exaggerating our daring escapade on the open sea.

Jennifer

Perhaps you've done something you think can't be undone. After all, Yardstick says we're expected to behave a certain way in life, and if we goof up in any way, we're in hot water. Let me tell you the story of Sydney Biddle-Barrow (a.k.a. the "Mayflower Madame"). Years ago a story broke that made Ms. Barrow—much to her consternation—a household word. She was accused of running a very high-class brothel, catering to some of the country's wealthiest and most well-known men. Now, with this kind of publicity, you can just give up and decide your life is over—especially if your picture is splashed all over the front page of newspapers. Sydney, on the other hand, didn't choose to buy any of Yardstick's propaganda. I remember seeing her at one of my New York City National Speakers Association functions. She was very visible, helping register attendees to the event. She also went on to speak professionally, a far cry from giving up because she'd previously made some poor choices in life.

Yardstick Exercise 4

It's so easy to label people based on our experiences and almost no knowledge of the individual/situation. Here's a good exercise. Look at some of the labels we attach to people on a daily basis, and see what our perception is. We've given you one to start with.

Example: Introverts: Slow   Extroverts: Loud mouths

1._____

2._____

3._____

4._____

It's human nature to pigeonhole people. Anyone who isn't like us, is not only different, but often, we feel they're wrong! We need to give others personal freedom to be in the world with their own personalities, while ignoring people who don't accept us for who we are. What Yardstick will never admit is that "it takes all kinds." We need diversity of knowledge, perception and experience to solve the problems of this world.

The Yardstick mentality wants to mandate only one way to process information and express personality. That, of course, means the rest of us may be compromising our basic nature, giving up our talents, passions or unique gifts that could better the world. Don't conform because your way is not the "accepted" preference of a boss, coworker or other dominant individual in your life. If your hear a different drummer, march away.

It isn't just the inner voice that says *sit up; hold your fork the right way; behave in a certain manner* that controls our choices. It might also be peer pressure to do drugs, have a drink or cheat on your spouse. These behavior choices are often the result of a strong message: if you want to hang with us, this is how it's done. Which fork to use or how to use a spoon for cocaine—all come from our keen awareness that there is an accepted right way and wrong way, and that the wrong way carries with it the painful repercussion of exclusion and rejection.

In fact, says Yardstick, what you wear, drive, do, who you know, where you've been, where you eat or what sorority you join are more important than what you are. Yardstick wants you to be in a constant state of acquisition, never satisfied with who you have.

We're not talking about a dissatisfaction that drives you to improvement, we're talking about a nagging feeling that you're not enough all by your lonesome. That sinking feeling that if you stop, you'll roll downhill into oblivion.

But what if you were valuable, even if you never did anything significant, never went anywhere interesting, never wore a designer label? What if you, as a human being, were enough? If that's true, then Yardstick is truly powerless. We're all surrounded by the message that certain achievements, clothing and specific possessions will make us feel more important. For a while they do, but in the end, peace of mind comes from knowing who you are and accepting that.

Yardstick Exercise 5

Ask yourself what emotions the following things elicit:

I own a new Porsche (BMW, Mercedes, Rolls).

I totaled the Porsche. I now drive a used '87 Cutlass.
I wear designer jeans and shirts.
There was a fire. I now wear clothes from the thrift shop.
I can go into any restaurant in town and order *a la carte*.
I buy my food with food stamps.
The person sitting next to me is a Rockefeller.
The person next to me is homeless.

We all have strong cultural messages that some things are good and some things mean we are less than okay. What if you could decide what you like based on what you enjoy, not on what other people told you would make you a better or more acceptable person?

What Is the Effect of Living Around Yardstick?

The effect is that no matter what you accomplish or own, you get a strong message it's not enough.

Jennifer

"So what?" That's what my first husband used to say to me—if I was lucky enough to get anything out of him—when I'd done something to be proud of. Now, as you're reading this you might be thinking to yourself, well I would've told that guy to go kiss his assets. Yet when you have Yardstick so in-grained in your psyche, you're so battered emotionally and psychologically, you can't respond flippantly like that. Instead, you keep looking for other ways to prove you're worthy of praise.

That particular "so what" I was remembering came

*when I got my first—and from what I can remember, also
my only—front-page story with a byline in the Nashville
Tennessean newspaper. We lived out in the Tennessee country-
side, really far away from everything. We had one of those
rural mailboxes at the end of a mile-long dirt road laced
with pebbles and potholes.*

*Sunday morning at the crack of dawn—or at least as
soon as I could safely assume they'd delivered the paper—I
went racing down the road to get it. I was so excited I could
hardly believe my story was going to be on the front page.
Such an honor! This for a woman whose past writing experience had been as society editor of a small-town newspaper.
But this was big time for me, and I was so excited I was almost hyperventilating when I raced back up the drive with
the front page in hand. I dashed into the house, summoned
my husband, showed him the story, and of course, you now
know his reply.*

*Did that make me angry? Nope. Yardstick just made
me want to try harder. Even more significantly, it made me
stop to think: was it such a big deal after all? I mean I
thought it was, but maybe I was just blowing the whole
thing to epic proportions and it was just another front-page
story. Guess I'd better try harder next time.*

Sally

*My brother didn't go to college, which in the suburbs
was the kiss of death for success. We all felt so sorry for him.
He had learning disabilities, and the school system gave him
limited opportunities for success. Our Yardstick for success left
him out of the picture. So, while I was scrambling up the corporate ladder, he was working blue-collar jobs. Then the*

layoffs and downsizing epidemic began, and while the col-
lege-educated members of the family were working part-time
jobs "between positions," he started a company in air condi-
tioning and heating.

I'm guessing it was a proud time, that weekend he in-
vited all his sisters to his four-bedroom home on the side of a
mountain to see the cathedral ceiling and indoor hot tub so-
larium. He was making at least two to three times as much
as we were, setting his own hours, doing his bookwork in the
hot tub and spending lots of quality time with his family.
My brother proved Yardstick wrong in the best way possi-
ble—by doing well outside the so-called rules. Oh, for the
record, his daughter graduated from college with top honors.

Where does Yardstick come from? The age of information
has brought with it higher expectations. Managers hear about
a competitor lowering prices or increasing service and demand
the same from you. They're seldom in touch with significant
reasons why one company can produce results and yours can't.
Many factors—such as procedure, red tape, budgets, laws,
capitalization, distribution, training—can all have an impact
on a company's effectiveness and bottom line.

Yardstick Exercise 6

Name a TV star you'd like to look (somewhat) like:

_____

Name a TV star you'd like your spouse to look like:

_____

These people are usually glamorous and beautiful. But very

---

few of us get to know the real person behind the glitz. The
truth is, these people are presented to us as real people, and
they're truly larger than life.

A man may see a glamorous model on TV, look across the
room at his middle-aged wife, and wonder why she can't
spruce herself up a bit to look like the model. Yet how many
men would like to spend $10,000 a month maintaining a
super model: haircut ($350); hair coloring ($500—a conserva-
tive estimate); plastic surgery ($20,000); cosmetics ($1000 a
month); shoes ($600 a pair); and on and on? Cher at fifty was
reported to have spent $100,000 in surgery to look like a mil-
lion bucks. That's a pretty good deal if you can come up with
the $100,000.

Likewise, a woman may wonder why her Mr. Right can't
pull in the old gut and give her that charming smile. Yet, how
many women would go for the cost of capped teeth and the
three hours a day at the gym Mr. Right would have to spend
to pull it together?

We see everything through airbrushed, three-angle light-
ing, makeup artists and touch-ups, and wonder why our world
can't be like that. It takes three weeks and a team of six people to make that model look so young, fresh and natural for a
fast few minutes. Our favorite article in a scandal paper was
one showing pictures of all the famous "babes" of Hollywood
with no make-up and dirty hair: you know, like the rest of us
look in the morning!

The glamorous reality we're comparing ourselves with
doesn't really exist. How many family problems are solved in
thirty minutes as they are in the TV sitcoms? How many people do you know who have hours a day to discuss their problems in endless dialogue?

Yardstick Exercise 7

In the 1960s they were still making judgments about which kids would do well in college and which shouldn't even try. They had a list of about fifty occupations and twenty colleges to choose from. Life has a funny way of changing in spite of us. Very few people even work in the field in which they received their degree.

List your area of degree or training and then list your job. Do it for five friends as well:

Job: *Area of study:*
Example: *Humor writer and speaker*   *Gerontology*

1._____

2._____

3._____

4._____

5._____

If we can work so far from our original field, perhaps we can find our future in a completely new area. We need to be willing to make our own path in life. Some people learned to do this early on in life, and others have needed a bit more time.

Yardstick Exercise 8

This is an exercise to help you predict the outcome of certain choices. It may also help you know what to do to find your own path. Start off with any pressure you're feeling to conform to a social Yardstick.

Take whatever you feel pressured to do: lose weight, travel more, work less. Now write out about ten lines in the following grid. It is important to go down to at least ten levels because as we work with this we're apt to get down to what we're afraid of and stop. Keep going until you find out where Yardstick violates who you are.

For example:

What if: I restrain myself around men. Then they'll feel comfortable around me.
If they feel comfortable around me, then they'll open up.
If they open up, then I'll open up.
If I open up, then they'll feel threatened.
If I threaten them, then I'll clam up.
If I clam up, then I'll feel rejected for being me.
If I feel rejected for being me, then I'll blame them.
If I blame them, then I'll have to take responsibility, too.
If I take responsibility, then I'll see that I was acting as someone I am not.
If I acted a pretend part or role, then I can't blame them for being threatened.

Here's where you break through!

If I can't blame them, then I need to be with men I don't threaten.
If I need to be with men I don't threaten, I need to meet smarter, more self-confident men.

If I need to meet smarter men, then I need to go to classes at the university or join business clubs.

How can you undo Yardstick's rule? You have to be clear on your own standards:

If I _____ *(dare to have what I want)*

then _____ *(this is what I'll have to do)*

If I _____

then _____

If I _____

then _____

If I _____

then _____

If I _____

then _____

If I _____

then _____

If I _____

then _____

If I _____

then _____

If I _____

then _____

Yardstick Exercise 9

If you're allowing yourself to be sickened into Yardstick thinking, then stop a minute and ask yourself why? In *Accelerated Learning for the 21st Century,* authors Colin Rose and Malcolm J. Nichol mention going five "whys" deep to really look at any issue. When dealing with Yardstick, it's a good wake-up call to ask why to see just how brainwashed we've become.

Jennifer played the game like this:

> *You can't be a successful motivational speaker and trainer.*
> Why?
> *Well, because you must have years of experience in the business.*
> Why?
> *Because that gives you the insight and personal expertise to coach others.*
> Why?
> *Because without those years in the business you can only fall back on your own trials and errors, and no one wants to hear about your life unless you can substantiate it with credibility.*
> Why?
> *Because people will only listen to you if they believe in you and your message.*

And on it goes.

The circle eventually gets back to the fact that I already had all I needed, as long as I quit listening to Yardstick.

Motivational speaker and author Anthony Robbins did the same thing. He published his own books and has sold hundreds of thousands of copies. Yet during one of his public seminars a man asked how to publish a book, and when Robbins told how he had self-published, the man said something to the effect of, "Yeah, but how can you publish a real book?" So the millions of dollars that Robbins has made with his books can't count unless a "real" publisher publishes them? What do *you* think?

The Yardstick "Why Game."

I want _____

but I can't have it because_____

Why? Why? Why? Why? Why?

Yardstick Exercise 10
Pressure gauge.

Make a list of all the pressures you suffer in order to conform. Rate your answers as important (score five points) down to not going to happen any time too soon (one point). Then add the name of the person this would please:

Pressure or Rule:	*Importance:*	*Person(s):*
Example: Stop smoking	4	Self, Boyfriend
1. _____		

2._____

3._____

4._____

5._____

Reminders

How Long Does it take to Have What You Want?

Often we get stuck believing if we're smarter or try harder we can get what we want immediately. Sometimes that's true, but more often than not, it involves a series of plateaus as we learn and grow to achieve what we want. We're desperate to move our business to the next level, and we do everything we can think of—including working fourteen-hour days—but to no avail. What's wrong with us?

Probably nothing. We have to be willing to keep on building, growing, providing the service, and often when we're not expecting it, the growth spurt will occur. Don't beat yourself up if you aren't achieving as rapidly as your college roommates, neighbors, cousins, or strangers you meet at parties who tell you how quickly they amassed their fortunes.

Most "overnight successes" have twenty years of experience and background to draw on. Actors and authors are excellent examples. It's just that no one else heard about their struggles except their families and close friends. Overnight can be a very long night!

Ad agencies want you to buy a product to look instantly younger, feel happier, make friends quicker, win your tennis game more powerfully, satisfy your family's appetites more rapidly, and on and on. They feed us a lust for instant gratification—right up Yardstick's alley—and when we buy into it, we have to feel dissatisfied with our own lives since we're trudging along with not even one instant, overnight success under our belt.

Even motivational stories lack appropriate real time; miracles often happen over ten to twenty years. In a book it's one chapter and "instant-presto" a miracle. Think of all the heroic stories of burn victims or paraplegics who've overcome their physical challenges and become entertainers or politicians or writers or even runners. In a book or TV movie the first quarter is about their tragedy, the next part is about their enlightenment and the last half is about the difference they're making with their courage. Have you ever been in a rehab center or burn ward? Success doesn't happen overnight. Overcoming these odds is more about tiny, unnoticeable benchmarks.

How many of us would be delighted and inspired to read that overcoming a physical accident or a bad marriage took the author twenty years? What if we wrote a motivational book called, *How to Cure Depression in Just Two Decades* or *The Thirty Year Diet Plan?*

No wonder we feel the weight of Yardstick all the time. Every place we go, people seem smarter, cuter, thinner and richer than we are. Yardstick works on imposing rigid rules about how to be successful in the world, as well as how we should act, think and look.

Remember, when it comes to physical appearances, there are only a few super models, and their photos are airbrushed. Anorexia and bulimia are the tragic results of telling women they aren't feminine unless they're size six or smaller. Women and girls buy into this Lie, instead of rejoicing in our thick thighs and round bottoms. Marilyn Monroe—sex symbol of the century—was a size fourteen! Yardstick's Lies about weight are killing us. Let's resist.

Get More Information.

Research and locate role models—people who live outside the expected norms. Read books or rent videos of the biographies of people such as Supreme Court judge Sandra Day O'Connor, Nobel Prize winner Marie Curie, anthropologist Margaret Mead. Seek out people who ignored the protocol and just did it a different way. Learn from them.

Your Action Plan

To make a plan, you need to gather more information. You need to know what areas of your life are under attack by Yardstick, and then you need to stick it to that Monster. You need to put up a defensive wall that says, "No!" Then you need to decide you'll go by your own standard.

☞ What else is possible if I had more time? Can I get up earlier, plan mealtimes better?

☞ What else is possible if I had more money? Can I save money by giving up junk food, alcohol, cigarettes, or doing odd jobs for cash?

☞ What if I'm wrong? Am I willing to change? Do I resist suggestions, do I say *no* first, am I full of reasons why new things won't work?

☞ Who can help me get what I need? What can I offer in

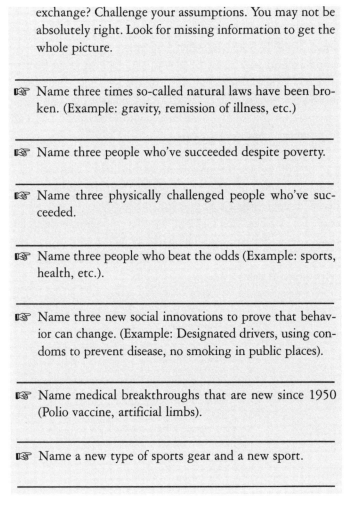

exchange? Challenge your assumptions. You may not be absolutely right. Look for missing information to get the whole picture.

☞ Name three times so-called natural laws have been broken. (Example: gravity, remission of illness, etc.)

☞ Name three people who've succeeded despite poverty.

☞ Name three physically challenged people who've succeeded.

☞ Name three people who beat the odds (Example: sports, health, etc.).

☞ Name three new social innovations to prove that behavior can change. (Example: Designated drivers, using condoms to prevent disease, no smoking in public places).

☞ Name medical breakthroughs that are new since 1950 (Polio vaccine, artificial limbs).

☞ Name a new type of sports gear and a new sport.

Summary

REVEAL the *Monster Lie* Yardstick and the damage It is trying to cause you. Don't concern yourself with appearances, designer labels and name brands. Your name is the only name brand you need. Instead, concentrate your life on what is good, what is pure and what will make a difference in the world around you. Every time you feel less important because you don't measure up, you need to ask yourself whose measuring stick you're using. Utilizing the measuring stick of the material world, society, Wall Street and Hollywood is a one-way ticket to low self-esteem.

It's time to ACT on your desires. Go back to school, learn a new skill, help someone else or ask for help. The RESULT is that you'll sort out all of this world's confusing messages and really discover what's important, what's lasting and what's true. Remember, don't spend another moment feeling less than others. You are as valuable as any movie star, as any corporate executive, as anyone is. It's up to you to recognize and celebrate this fact.

CHAPTER TEN
The Monster Lie Stuck-in-the-Mud

The truth Stuck-in-the-Mud doesn't want you to know:
If you want results, you're the one who has to change.

As we REVEAL Stuck-in-the-Mud you'll see It wants you to use up your time and energy trying to make other people act the "right way." Is someone drinking too much? Hide their beer cans. Is someone spending too much money? Hide the credit cards. This Monster wants you to get so involved with other people that you forget to take action for yourself. It's time to ACT. The RESULT of allowing others to deal with the consequences of their own bad choices is that you'll have an entire life to focus on your own plans, on what's important to you.

Meet Stuck-in-the-Mud

We can't change others, but Stuck-in-the-Mud tells you that you must spend a tremendous amount of energy trying to do just that. In the meantime, you must suffer quietly, hoping others will one day change their behavior. After all, if your time is invested in worrying about the actions of others and trying to manipulate them, then you don't have to take any responsibility or ownership for what's happening in your own life.

Of course, if instead you stop trying to change others and take full responsibility for what's happening in your life, then no one can have control over you. And that's a powerful place to be!

Stuck-in-the-Mud's Voice

Stuck-in-the-Mud speaks to you in a gravelly, syrupy voice that is always being projected over someone else's dialogue, loudly proclaiming the latest irritation or information:

I can't believe I have to wait for this guy to get me the report.
She makes me so mad.
He really hurts my feelings.
No one helps me around here.
I'm just furniture to you.
She's a witch, but what can I do?
We'll be late. He always makes us late.
She doesn't know how furious that makes me.
You're giving me a headache.
You're driving me crazy.
The people in this company are so negative.
I'd love to come, but I have to take care of _
My employees/my children keep me from what I want.

Who do you believe has control over you? Is that person the one who refuses to change, or is it you?

Stuck-in-the-Mud Exercise 1

List here the things you say about others who keep you involved:

1. _____

2. _____

3. _____

4. _____

Now what would happen if you could just ignore these
people for a short while and put all that energy into having
your own dreams come true? It's time to find out who Stuck-
in-the-Mud is and kick It out of your life.

Visualizing Stuck-in-the-Mud

Stuck-in-the-Mud is a prickly, sticky-looking porcupine
whose quills are always "stuck in the mud." It is usually
bogged down in the muck and mire of everyone else's problems, so Stuck-in-the-Mud can't move. The filth of others is so
much a part of It that Stuck-in-the-Mud never knows where
It ends and others begin. Stuck-in-the-Mud forgets to take
care of Itself so often, most people actually think Stuck-in-the-
Mud is a ball of mud and goo instead of what It is.

How Does Stuck-in-the-Mud Limit You?

"What have you done so far to change the situation you're
in?"

This is a powerful question and one not always greeted with a smile. Many of us would rather complain than do something about a situation. Time and again people will say how frustrated they are because so-and-so treats them badly, won't change his or her behavior, or how annoying a certain behavior is. So what? That is to say, "So what have you done about it?"

Logically, we go into any relationship, any friendship, with high expectations. As we truly get to know people, we often discover our initial impressions were incorrect. They aren't the people we thought they were. What do we do? We let people know our intent to have our needs met. If it's clear this isn't going to happen, then we should *vamoose*.

Stuck-in-the-Mud Exercise 2

Who takes up most of your time—other than small children who need attention? Who are you always reacting to, instead of living your life?

1. _____

2. _____

3. _____

4. _____

5. _____

What if you started looking for ways to spend energy on your future and stopped getting in the middle of others' lives. We really do have a choice, but we don't always realize it.

Facing the Monster Stuck-in-the-Mud: Our Stories

Jennifer

First she pulled my garbage bag from the compactor room and dumped it in front of my door. Then she began leaving hate mail taped to my door. Suffice it to say, I figured out she didn't like me much. I tried everything from talking to her, to complaining about her. Anything to find out why she disliked me. If I was on an elevator and she saw me, she would wait for another elevator.

This woman, who was my neighbor for years, was quite a challenge. I smiled, said good morning, and finally woke up to the fact that I must look like the first grade teacher she hated. For whatever reasons, she chose to put her energy into hating me. I decided right then not to try to do anything at all. I simply lived my life and when I ran into her from time to time, she immediately jumped off the elevator as if I had a wildly infectious disease. But that was her problem. Since we can't change people, please don't invest any of your energy and ego into trying.

Sometimes our inclination is to wait a little longer to see if we're possibly mistaken; to see if we can, in fact, change the other person. We're apt to be more understanding because of mitigating circumstances right at this particular moment, or to hope someone will give us what we need without our insisting on it. What doesn't work is assuming others will change without a struggle.

You must be clear on what you need, hold your ground or leave. Staying and whining, staying and suffering, nagging, pleading, begging: it not only demeans you, it doesn't work.

217

Bending your boundaries should never be an option.

What most people do is linger and hope. They volunteer to become victims and then talk about all the time they've already invested. Cut your losses and realize no one has to change for you, nor you for them. Not to say life is not a series of compromises, but real changes, those that require people to alter how they behave, don't happen at our bidding.

If you say you love a job, partner, neighborhood, or store all except for this "one thing," listen to yourself. "One thing" is not acceptance. It is a lobbying effort to make them in our image. This is not where any of us should put our energies.

Jennifer

There's an old story that's been around a long time and is highly significant because it teaches us that we have choices. Two brothers grew up with a dad who was in prison for armed robbery and murder. One of the young men finished college and was teaching at a university. He made a sterling example of his life. The other was in prison.

When interviewed, both gave the same answer for why their lives had turned out the way they did: "I had no choice, with a father like that." One used his dad as an excuse, and became the victim. The other used his dad as the catalyst to propel himself forward.

Stuck-in-the-Mud will tell you that you should spend all your energy trying to change other people. It wants you to believe that the key to your happiness is in somebody else's pocket.

"If only my boss were reasonable, my spouse passionate, the government effective, my sister sober, then . . . ." Stuck-in-the-Mud wants you neck deep into other people's lives so you never have to tend to your own. If you spend all your energy trying to change others and the world around you, then you can avoid personal responsibility for real change. Employees not dependable? Complain about it. Spouse an alcoholic? Good. Then let everyone know how hard that makes your life and how much you have to suffer. After all, what else can you do? Don't change your own actions. Don't get your own life together. Wait for others to change first.

If you want to suffer for a lifetime, by all means, rescue the person with bad behavior, cover up their bad choices, and pay for their consequences with your own resources. Never let them grow into full adulthood. The payoff? You never get a life, but you can apply for sainthood.

Stuck-in-the-Mud Exercise 3

What can you do right now before others change? Example: Choose to be in a good mood. Choose to let go of resentment.

Now list changes you can make every day: eating habits, sleeping habits, tone of voice, attitude, etc.

1._____

2._____

3._____

4._____

5._____

It seems to be human nature to blame other people when we don't like the way things are working out. We don't take responsibility for the outcome of our actions or lack of actions. Blame is the oldest game there is. It is the base of all conflict. It is just so much easier to hope others will change their basic nature and take care of things. The problem is, that leaves us standing around waiting for something to happen. How much better is it to simply start the ball rolling?

Jennifer

An acquaintance of mine, a bright woman, stays with the same man she's been with for the last twenty years. Not because she's in love with him, but because, she says, she has given him the best years of her life. But shouldn't the best years be those ahead of her?

Now he has to suffer with her anger and take care of her. Do we even need to talk about it to see what's wrong with this picture? Let it go, give it up, stop putting energy into revenge, anger, grief and excuses. There is more to life!

The Lie of Stuck-in-the-Mud is that your value in Life is to change others first; that your past will continue to replay itself into the future. We're waiting for others to change so we can begin our change process. Others, however, aren't operating by our schedule. But what if we could see every day as a brand new day? What if we have a clean slate and no excuses for not having good things in our life? What if we don't have to unpack our old baggage? What if we're accountable to create each day from scratch? What if we set the rules anew and lived that way? Is there any reason why we can't begin changing age-old rules?

People do it all the time. Do you collect the pot of money

in the middle of the Monopoly board when you land on Free Parking? If so, you're creating your own rules. In the official Monopoly rule book if someone lands on luxury tax and pays seventy-five "dollars" into the kitty, that goes to the bank, not the middle. If you land on Free Parking you don't get to keep it. But most of us scratch that rule, play the one that is more fun for us, and don't worry about it at all.

Sally attended a women's conference with Suzanne Sommers, Erica Jong and Gloria Steinham as guest authors. Someone in the audience asked Ms. Steinham why we were just now hearing about co-dependency. Was it a new disease? Her answer, "No, it's been around, [but] in the '50s it was called accepted housewife behavior."

Stuck-in-the-Mud Exercise 4

List new rules that would make your life easier.

Example: everybody over the age of twelve has to take a turn cooking dinner; no one is allowed to make fun of your artwork, etc.

1. _____

2. _____

3. _____

4. _____

5. _____

These new rules may not make you any friends. Nobody

likes change, but people will adapt. The key is that you stop waiting for people to notice how wonderful you are so they'll be inspired to change or help you or stop drinking or start working. Now is the day of the new order, *your* order! Now is the day to change the rules so you can have your life back.

Often people talk of unanswered prayers and say God didn't answer their pleas. When asked if they expected those prayers to be answered, the usual answer is: "Well, not really." How can we have prayers answered, better feelings, good results, peace, new job opportunities, if we don't expect we'll get what we want?

Please don't use that old excuse: "If I don't expect anything, I won't get disappointed." Ah, but you're expecting something. You're expecting to be disappointed, unhappy, complacent, and not to get what you want. Change your expectations, and continue to expect only the best.

Mary Baker Eddy, founder of the Christian Science Church and author of *Science and Health* always expected her patients to be healed, always expected positive results, despite tremendous controversy from the clergy.

In business, we're apt to let others determine our success. In big corporations, so much of what we do ties into others' behavior. Some of the best business practices occur when someone says, "I know this is the way it was always done, but I'm going to change it." You're the only one you *can* change. Why should you be the one to change? The answer is this: because you want more in life. You have vision and hope and nobody can take that from you.

Why Is it Always *Me* Who Has To Change?

You don't! You only have to be the one to change if you

want new results or better relationships or a better life. The person who is willing to change is the person who wants more in life.

Do you want to stop being offended by know-it-all relatives? Want to go to college? Lose weight? Stop stressing out over your boss? Learn French? Learn how to forgive insensitive people or those who betray you?

What must you do to have what you want? Let go of trying to please the relatives and get their approval. Go to the library, call a college for student assistance, barter with a French student for lessons, talk to your boss or change jobs. Author Wayne Dyer reminds us that conflict cannot survive without our cooperation. We can create the change that does away with the conflict; we get to choose! Remember, you can wait until somebody gives you more money, better clothes, a bigger house, an exercise room in your own home—or you can start to change now. People can adapt to each other, they can compromise, but they can't change their basic character. They don't have to. Don't expect others to change. They might, but don't count on it. Especially if those people are unstable, highly emotional or have a pattern of conflict at every turn. Turn away from those people. Be proactive with your energy to create the life you want.

The most amazing power we possess is being in charge: how we're reacting, how much say we have in our lives. You can choose not to get all tangled up in other people's craziness. You don't have to defend yourself. Just walk away—quickly.

What is the cost of tying your life up with other people who must change first before you get peace and happiness? It is the same as expecting interest on a savings account when all your money is under your mattress. If you don't put your money and resources in a position to grow, they can't. There are no bonus points in Heaven for forgetting to use your gifts. There are no "do over" days in life.

Sally

My stepfather was a gifted carpenter, but he worked as a flight engineer. He hated the people he worked for, hated the hours, and he hated himself for not being smart enough to get a better job. He kept hoping his boss would be kinder and more thoughtful. He always wished his parents had been more loving. (Of German descent, they actually put coal in his stocking one year at Christmas to teach him a lesson.) He waited and waited. He complained and complained. His friends kept saying, "Leave, start your own woodworking business." But he wasn't about to give that hated boss the satisfaction of knowing he had drummed him out.

So my stepfather had three heart attacks, had to retire early and then died of his fifth heart attack several years later. The good news is that at the very end of his life he began doing things for himself—things he liked—instead of waiting for others to change. The cost of staying where you hate to be and complaining as you wait for others to change is that it can actually kill you.

Jennifer

When I was waiting for my first marriage to get miraculously better, I had a variety of physical problems. I was hospitalized for colitis several times. Once my doctor came into my hospital room, shut the door and told me I had to make some changes in my life. At the rate I was going, he warned, I would end up with something more serious, such as colon cancer. Perhaps he was trying to scare me into action.

Unfortunately, his advice didn't help. I stuck out the situation, partially because I couldn't see the options. If you're taught the ocean is terrible, and you've never ventured from land—never even seen a boat or a swimmer—you'd be hard pressed to imagine leaving the safety of land and getting in that wet stuff. You have no vision, no realm of possibility to hang that vision on.

Consequently, it's imperative that we see and understand there are options, and many of them. Start with small pictures if need be, and expand your vision slowly. Dare to imagine. No one has to know your visions and fantasies. But it'll be difficult for them to become realities unless you can imagine them actually happening.

The way my marriage ended was simple: he walked out with a suitcase in hand and that was that. As I waited day by day to die, it dawned on me that I didn't like my life, but I was still breathing, still functioning, and that meant there were many other possibilities—visions—out there for me. I began to rebuild my life a day at a time. Seeing yourself as an agent for change is vital, along with deciding you'll absolutely not stay where you are when there are so many other places you can be. They key is not to let the Stuck-in-the-Mud monster control your thinking.

Stuck-in-the-Mud Exercise 5

What is it you've always wanted to do? What talents or gifts did you have as a child that have been brushed aside? Playing an instrument, playing a sport, painting, collecting stamps or telling jokes?

Write down five things that you've stopped doing because someone else is or has stopped you from doing them, sometimes by taking up your time, and often by disapproving.

Now write down who is stopping you and why.

Example:

Thing you love: *Go to funny movies and laugh loudly*
Who is stopping you?   *My mother-in-law*

Thing you love:_____

Who is stopping you?_____

Thing you love:_____

Who is stopping you?_____

Thing you love:_____

Who is stopping you?_____

Thing you love:_____

Who is stopping you?_____

Thing you love:_____

Who is stopping you?_____

It's been said, "Most people die in their twenties, they just wait until their sixties to be buried." There are tricks that can help you take charge. Remember that waiting for others to change is putting off your future and your fortune.

Stuck-in-the-Mud Exercise 6
Just a sample.

When you think about your life, are there things that seem to be slipping past you? Are there opportunities you can't take because of previous responsibilities and commitments? Here's an exercise to help you recover some of what seems to be passing you by.

List what you would like to do:

_____

Next, identify how that would make you feel:

_____

Now see if there is some part (perhaps only a small part) you can have, or work toward, right now:

_____

List in detail what you would have to do to make part of this a reality:

1._____

2._____

3._____

4._____

5._____

This is not compromising as much as it's refusing to let your current life cut you out of joy and discovery. You can have a small nugget of gold while you're waiting for the mother lode. Don't postpone joy, celebration or getting a piece of the action. Increase your reality by giving yourself good things

SALLY FRANZ & JENNIFER WEBB

now!

Too many people act like spoiled children. If they can't have it all right now, the way they want it, it isn't worth having. Things may not work out to be your one-hundred-percent ideal dream. So consider this type of activity as the dress rehearsal. Many people who go to France eat at French restaurants months before the trip just to practice their French with the waiters.

Stuck-in-the-Mud Exercise 7
Take Responsibility.

Decide on the desired result. Fill in name of desired result:

Example: *get a refund on a warranty.*

Now list the names and numbers of people who can make it happen:

Example: *store manager, customer service department, company headquarters representative.*

Stuck-in-the-Mud Exercise 8

Make a specific list of what you want in the next five years.

Then list what or who you used as an excuse for not getting what you wanted in the past. These excuses are now forbidden!

Make a list of specific steps you will take to see the results you want.

_____

List when you will begin each step

_____

List all the resources, experts, friends, people who can help, and call them, beginning with two calls today.

_____

Anticipate everything that won't go your way, and be prepared: people who're angry that you aren't paying attention to their own dilemmas, people telling you that you're selfish; people saying you can't reach your dreams.

_____

_____

Plan to keep moving forward until you get what you want, no matter what!

Stuck-in-the-Mud Exercise 9

Think of all the things that are new inventions made by people who stopped listening to others' negativity. Think of how many of these new things wouldn't exist if their inventors were caught up in the manipulation of others. What if the inventors were so busy rescuing others they forgot to get a patent or backers? You have marvelous work to do. Stop getting weighed down in the mud!

Name all the new innovations you can:

New office equipment since 1960:_____

New music style:_____

New kitchen equipment:_____

New toy for kids:_____

New medical procedure:_____

New song on the radio you really like:_____

New authors, books, movies:_____

New car design or feature:_____

Do you have new beliefs? Are there some beliefs you should let go of? Be willing to be wrong so that you can have your dreams. Remember not to get stuck with an old plan or idea that's no longer relevant. Be willing to be yelled at when everybody else wants you to do things the same old way. Say *no,* smile, and go about your business.

Are people angry that you're moving on? If necessary, go to the library, or to the backyard to get away from others who expect you to give up your new dreams so that you can do things for them. Most likely they're perfectly capable of doing things for themselves. Some people have a nasty habit of being waited on. Every healthy child over ten—and that means grown-ups—can feed and dress themselves. Most can do the laundry and cook as well.

Stuck-in-the-Mud Exercise 10
Check your intent level.

What do you really want more than anything?

_____

How can you have that legally?

_____

If you had it, how would it help others?

What is stopping you?

How could you have some of this right now?

Is there something else you need to do to have this?

Will it be worth it, and do you really want this one thing more than the inconvenience it will take to get it?

Generally, we're fine caring for others, but we feel selfish and guilty when we care for ourselves. We need to find a balance, and that only comes from taking care of ourselves as we would for a loved one.

Reminders

You Do the Math!

It may feel as if you're the sum total of the things that happened to you, but everyone has calamity and craziness in their path. It's the choices you make and the meaning you give those incidents that shape your life. You're dealt a hand. Maybe it's not a good one, but you can always exchange some cards and throw away the ones that don't match your vision. Even if the only thing you can change at first are your reactions and attitude, don't let others rob you of your belief in yourself.

Whatever is the root of your unrest, you need to assess the damage. Take stock of your resources, abilities and drive. Pick up and get back on the path. Remember, if it were easy, everybody would have done it by now!

What Some Great Minds Have to Say

Vive la Différence.

Read David Keirsey and Marilyn Bates, *Please Understand Me*. It is all about Carl Jung's work and the work of Myers and Briggs discussing personality typing. The most important thing you get from their work is that everybody has ways to process information and decisions. If they differ from yours, that doesn't make them wrong. Keirsey and Bates have done an excellent job explaining how to value differences. It's worth a read. The important thing is that you be yourself and celebrate that.

In order to move forward, we must be willing to take chances, take ownership, not wait for others to create changes for us, and to look foolish along the way. Otherwise we're staying in our safe little environments, unwilling to venture out for fear of making a mistake.

Stuck-in-the Mud is one Monster who really doesn't like to go away. The best thing to do is regularly review your plans. If anything you want is slow in coming, you may ask if you're waiting for someone to change before you act; or are you specific enough in your plan, or have you analyzed what's holding you back? Now take action, any little action. Just get going. Preempt fate. Even if it's as small as writing sticky notes to yourself and plastering them all over your house as reminders that where you are is a stopping post, not the end of the line! Even if you just cut your cigarettes in half to slow down your smoking on the way to quitting. Start now with some small step.

Go Around the Negative People.

Remember, your true limitations have nothing to do with someone's perceptions of your limitations. Many of the things we've done were carried out despite severe warnings. "It's the worst mistake you've made in your life," was one comment Jennifer got when she started her own business. "It'll never work," and other similar words of doom were given to both of us regarding our businesses, our book, and other related projects.

If you spend any of your time worrying about what other people believe you're capable of doing, you'll be lucky to get out the door in the morning. Don't try to change those folks, just move on around them. In spite of them, enjoy the power and freedom it creates for you. Loosen up your thinking muscles. We're often so submerged in the negative we forget all of the progress others have made that we can also make. To get to be a believer again, dwell, meditate, concentrate on the many amazing things that are taking place all around you.

Your Action Plan

☞ Who are the most significant people in your life?

☞ How many of those people are under the age of twelve (or even six)?

All the rest are capable people able to get their own meals, do laundry, get up on time, write notes, call when late, be considerate of others, stay sober, return borrowed items intact.

Now that you'll have a great deal of time not caretaking for capable people, list three things you'd like to do or learn:

1. _____

2. _____

3. _____

Summary

Stuck-in-the Mud wants you to be mesmerized by everyone else's problems. Should you be worried about their hurts, their problems, or their anxieties? You can care, but don't try to fix them. It's not selfish; it's taking care of yourself. The truth about Stuck-in-the Mud is It wants you to be so involved with the problems of other people that you feel as if you no longer actually exist. The more you do that for others the less they will respect you; the more they will demand of you. It's a lousy system!

So let's get real. **REVEAL** that Stuck-in-the-Mud wants to gobble up your every waking minute and then **ACT**. What action should you take? Untangle what is others' responsibilities and what is yours. Did they forget their homework? Why are *you* driving back to school to get it? They'll have to resolve this themselves. Is an adult confused and lonely? They need therapy, not to be using up all your time when they have no intention of ever helping you, or caring about you, or helping themselves. Tell them you love them, tell them to go to therapy, tell them to go to church or temple but by all means tell them good-bye.

Note: If you reject Stuck-in-the Mud, the **RESULT** is you'll find those adults who were dependent on you will be annoyed, if not outright hostile. Hold firm. All that time you spent rescuing others will now be available for following your own dreams! It's definitely worth the energy and frustrations it takes to get to a place where you can take care of yourself.

CHAPTER ELEVEN

The Monster Lie Clairvoyant

The truth Clairvoyant doesn't want you to know:
If I have to guess what you're thinking, then I'll probably get it wrong.

We're going to REVEAL Clairvoyant, who wants you to be offended when people don't anticipate your needs, read your mind or understand you the first time. Instead we'll show you how to ACT to get the results you want by implementing smarter communication skills. The RESULT is you'll waste less energy feeling frustrated and will be able to reach people much more effectively to get what you really want.

Meet the Monster Clairvoyant

"Notice anything different?" How many men have had terror strike their hearts when the women they love walk into the room and make them guess which addition or change is new? Every guy is thinking, "I've got about two thousand chances to be wrong here, and one chance to be right." This is a game where the woman thinks she's testing the man's love. The problem is this test isn't measuring love, devotion and faithfulness. This game tests a man's ability to notice details. Usually the man who can pass this test will also remind you there's dust on top of the refrigerator, warn you the expiration date is almost up on the milk and let you know when you have gained an extra ten pounds. Is this the behavior you want to encourage?

Clairvoyant's Voice

Clairvoyant likes you to think everyone who cares about you should know what you want before you ask them. Subdued and demure, Clair's voice almost purrs when reminding you:

> *If you really cared about me, you'd know what I like.*
> *You don't have to say a word. I know what you're thinking.*
> *You know how I feel about that already.*
> *Don't you remember what I like to drink?*
> *You know I hate marigolds.*
> *Pearls? Who wears pearls anymore?*
> *You call this a business proposal?*
> *Why do I have to tell you everything?*

Clairvoyant Exercise 1

Where and when do you expect others to read your mind? Make a list of who you expect to read your thoughts, and what you expect them to know:

1. _____

2. _____

3. _____

4. _____

5. _____

Visualizing Clairvoyant

Clairvoyant looks harmless, but It can be dangerous. Clairvoyant resembles a flighty, transparent blue and pink butterfly. It flutters about making a lot of noise accomplishing nothing. Clairvoyant is indignant if you don't know what It's thinking. It wants to encourage you to be very annoyed if people can't read your mind.

Clairvoyant will tell you: "If people really loved you, cared for you and were smarter, they would understand you." People should know what you want, what you mean and when to do things for you. If they don't give you what you want, they must not be very interested in you. They must not be as committed as you are to the job.

For bonus points, Clairvoyant urges you to be as vague as possible when making a request. This will really prove how much other people care about you. Say things such as: "I want this paper to look professional this time!" Or: "If you don't know why I'm upset, then I'm not going to tell you!"

Clairvoyant is a part of our culture. Our society is moving so very fast that we shortcut everything, including our language. Now if we were a homogeneous population, perhaps more like Japan, words would have much the same meaning, and we'd no doubt share the same values and work ethics. But in this day and age in America, we have as many definitions as we have cultural backgrounds.

How many is that? Sally was once hired to create an advertising poster for a park in Brooklyn, New York. She suggested using the languages of the neighborhood groups as a border for the poster. There were twenty-three languages and dialects represented around one park. Today, even in the Midwest, there are people from all over the world in the smallest of towns. You can't assume people understand you—or that you understand them—without talking it out.

How Does Clairvoyant Limit You?

We all carry our personal dictionary around in our head. It isn't words according to Webster, it's words according to *us*. The problem comes when we forget that very simple words have very different meanings and cultural weight. Add to that, family upbringing, regional dialects and accents. You could place bets how few people mean the same thing when they communicate using even simple phrases.

After she moved to New York City, Jennifer kept trying to figure out what she was doing to make the grocery clerk give her such funny looks. Coming from rural America, she kept telling him she didn't need a sack; she would carry the item. No one knew what she was referring to, since in New York you refer to a bag, not a sack. In the Midwest people often ask for pop, not a diet Coke or Pepsi. We all speak different kinds of English. These are such simple, innocuous examples—nothing that involves the real stress we often feel when we don't communicate correctly. *USA Today* cites poor communication skills as one of the main financial drains on corporations. We aren't clear, people don't understand, and mistakes are made that are costly and time-consuming.

At work, for example, exactly what time of day do you mean when you ask your assistant to bring you a report by the "end of the day?" Is that your end of the day, considering you often leave at 4:00 p.m. during the summer to get in a game of golf? Or is it your assistant's time of day? He leaves at 7:00 p.m. because he covers the switchboard until the building closes. What does it mean for someone to come to work "on time?" That might mean on the dot of 9:00 a.m. to one individual, 9:15 a.m. to another and 7:30 a.m. to yet another.

Amazing, isn't it, how easy it is to miscommunicate the most obvious things. Not only must we work on communicating with the expectation that people might not understand us, but we can't expect people simply to *know* how we're feeling, no matter how often we send cues and clues instead of clear messages:

"I've got a headache." Meaning: Can't he see I'm not up to finishing that report?

"No, nothing's wrong. I just don't want to talk." Meaning: When will he realize he forgot my birthday?

"There's nothing good on this menu!" Meaning: When is she going to wake up to the fact I hate going to this place for dinner?

Even if we know people so intuitive they often seem to read our mind, we can't expect it to work always. So we must be responsible for telling people what we think, feel, need, etc.

In our interpersonal life we often carry around the myth that if people don't know what we want, then they don't really care or love us. How many of us have heard—or said the following upon being asked why someone was upset: "Well, if you don't know, I'm not going to tell you!"

When you're a person who feels very deeply, it's hard to imagine that anyone can be so heartless as not to know what's upsetting you. The problem is that some people aren't wired to feel that deeply—at least not about the things you care about. They can care about you and not know what you need, even after twenty years.

Clairvoyant Exercise 2

List three things you wish the world knew about you without having to tell them:

Example: I *don't like being called Mrs. Franz. I'm happily divorced and Mrs. bothers me. Use Ms.*

1. _____

2. _____

3. _____

How are others supposed to find out your needs? Even if others wanted to help you, they can't if you don't give them enough information or the tools. Telling people what you want without anger is the best way to ensure that you get it.

Imagine you and your spouse/significant other are stuck in traffic and you're running late for the opera. To you, it may feel like the end of the world. You're upset to miss the opening, and you can already feel the embarrassment and humiliation of coming in late. You'd actually even prefer not to go if you have to enter late. Your spouse views this very differently. He couldn't care less about what other people in the audience think. You feel the weight of the world; he feels the weight of a feather. Who's right? Both people. You feel what you feel. No one can help how they feel. All you can do is modify your outward reaction.

By the way, he may feel passionately about certain things that you don't. Say *you* backed over his golf clubs, and they now look like some futuristic sculpture. He might actually sit down and cry. You're thinking, big deal, so we go to the sporting goods store and buy new ones. He should even be happy he's getting a new set.

Clairvoyant wants us to demand that others feel the way we do, and then, of course, they should know what to do and say. We all place different values on everyday things. Yet we all function as if we're working from the same set of directions and the very same dictionary with a standard definition for every word. Not only do we have our own definitions; each definition is weighted and rated as to importance for survival. To some, being *neat* means there's a path between the clutter wide enough for two people to pass each other if they both turn sideways. To another, *neat* means clear surfaces and one magazine on the coffee table.

Facing the Monster Clairvoyant: Our Stories

Sally

I wanted to finish school, but I never told my husband. He really thought folding diapers was fulfilling for me. How would he know? I never told him my dreams. When I finally enrolled in classes, he was really surprised. I thought he should know my secret dreams. I was wrong. There may be no support for your ambitions, but you have to say them out loud anyway.

Jennifer

Several years ago, I planned a half-surprise birthday party for a man I was dating. Because of his spectacular view of Manhattan from the New Jersey side of the Hudson, I wanted the party in his home, and because it would be more of a surprise if he didn't know the number of people coming, I told him I wanted to invite over only two couples to his home for dinner. I asked him to please make sure the house was very clean because guests would be coming over and when I'd get there Saturday I needed a fair amount of time to cook. Actually—since I do very little cooking—I needed a very large amount of time to shop for prepared foods and get everything heated up.

I must have reminded him ten times of the importance of picking up his home. He assured me it was cleaner and more in order than usual—all ready for a party. You can imagine my horror when I got there. Clothes everywhere and an amazing amount of junk on the floor, on the tables, everywhere you looked. But, the sink was cleared of dishes, the comforter was thrown over the bed, and the coffee table had been cleaned. To him this was "clean." To me, it was hideous. It took me something like three hours just to make it presentable for the thirty or so surprise guests who showed up later.

Sally

Once I attended a seminar at Columbia University. The students explained a test they'd developed to help social workers decide whether or not older people were competent to stay in their own homes. They'd prepared questions to check off, including: Must say the last seven presidents' names starting with today and going backward; has a clean house; keeps dishes relatively clean, and the like.

I pointed out that if, as a definition reference, I were to use my own standards of housekeeping as a working mother with two kids, nobody but I would be in the old age home. If they used some of my uptight friends' standards, we would all be in the home. To judge someone's competence on arbitrary and relative definitions is not only subjective, it is unproductive and a waste of valuable time.

What we have to do is painstakingly explain what to us seems so incredibly obvious. Most of us suffer fools lightly. We expect that either other people are bluffing to annoy us or con us, or that they're really stupid. Yet you wouldn't necessarily expect someone from another country to know what you were saying if you spoke your language to him.

If you storm around this world angry that people don't put the same importance on things that you do, you'll be mad a great deal of the time. When we live life as if everyone is in sync with our definitions and values, we set ourselves up for failure.

Time and again in the work place we've seen an employees ask a legitimate questions and have a manager say, "Go away and figure it out. I'm not here to teach you." That's as bad as when a teacher—when asked how to spell a word— tells the student to look it up in the dictionary. If you don't know enough of the correct spelling, how can you look it up?

The best way to avoid surprises in life is to be as specific as possible in the beginning. That goes for everything from renting a house to falling in love; from buying a car to having surgery. Without being specific, we run into the danger of people assuming, filling in the blanks with their own autobiographies.

A friend of ours had eye surgery to cure an infection. Afterwards she was surprised that her vision wasn't much better. Someone had told her that improved sight was possible with this surgery. "Oh," said her doctor, "I just assumed you wanted the same prescription. Some people get so used to wearing glasses; I didn't know you wanted vision correction as well as repair work." Most of us assume that others think the way we do. It is safer to assume that no one thinks the exact way you do.

One of the main reasons we may assume everyone understands us is that we often prefer to avoid confrontation. We'd feel awkward asking a loved one, "Okay, exactly what do you mean by saying, 'I love you?' Do you need me or want me or love me like you can't live without me? Speak up, boy!" Similarly, if someone asks us if we know what they mean on a certain topic, we often say yes. Sometimes we think we do know, but more often than not, we agree and nod our heads to avoid looking stupid. We rationalize it's probably not that important. So just nodding and mumbling is an easy way to get by.

Clairvoyant Exercise 2:

Describe a perfect meal:

_____

_____

Now describe it to the person who must cook the meal:

_____

_____

Did you include recipes? Did you explain where to buy ingredients? There is more to a perfect meal than candlelight. The entire meal must be created. If you're a chef, then you would probably be able to fill up a chapter of instructions. If not, you probably have taken a lot for granted, such as cooling the glassware and heating the plates.

Jennifer

Years ago I used to present a technical seminar. Vividly, I remember one day asking the audience if there was anyone who didn't know what "paradigm" was. No one raised a hand, so I continued. About fifteen minutes later, I was talking about a completely different subject, and a woman raised her hand. She said, "I think they're all lying." Now I was pretty baffled, and I politely asked her to what she was referring. She explained that when I asked everyone if they knew what paradigm was, she hadn't known, but she didn't want to be the only one asking.

Don't guess. Don't speculate on what you think someone is thinking. Well-known marketer Nancy Koehn was quoted in *Fortune Small Business Magazine* advising small business owners to spend an afternoon with colleagues, mulling over key questions: Whom do you most want to appeal to, and how are you communicating with them? How do you define your relationship with your target customer? How are you at maintaining that relationship?

Sally

"Okay," I thought, "make a note of this. When driving there is only one kind of flashing light worse than the one in your rearview mirror. It's the one on your dashboard."
I'd rented a car in the south of France to drive along the

serpentine roads of the Riviera. I stopped at a place with a spectacular view to take pictures. Right after that I noticed the lights on the dashboard were flashing. I calmed myself down from an all-out panic to a pulse-controlled frenzy. Pulling off the narrow road onto a three-inch shoulder, blind to anyone coming around the corner and nestled under an ancient hanging rock that looked tired of staying up, I began to rummage the glove compartment. I started pulling everything out of the glove box the way you'd rip your clothes off if you'd stepped in a pile of red ants.

At last I found the owner's manual—written, of course, in French. The sum total of my French is: bouquet, Chanel, French fries, French kiss and French toast. It never occurred to me that anyone would rent me a brand new car and let me drive down the road with the wrong driver's manual. After playing the Wheel of Fortune version of turning over every button and switch, it turned out that I had left the emergency brake up a teensy bit.

Now it occurs to me to check for owners' manuals. Lots of things occur to me. I may seem paranoid, picky and uptight, but I have fewer and fewer unpleasant surprises in life by being very clear up front and never assuming.

Clairvoyant Exercise 3
Loop de loop.

One of the best ways to find out if the people in your life are understanding you is to create an information loop. It is important to know that people have a very short (in seconds) attention span. They tune in and out all day long.

For example, If you suspect that someone is drifting off while you're giving them directions, the best thing is to say, "Often I'm not clear in what I say. I'm not sure if I included all of the directions in order. Would you read back to me, or share with me what you heard, so that I can make sure I gave you the correct information?"

But wait, you say, it's not my fault if they're dropping off and losing information. Well, it is and it isn't. After all, you're the one talking. If you're droning or vague, you might want to take some ownership of the fact that your communication skills may be lacking. It's always best to assume it was your lack of communication. Because you can only change yourself anyway. You're the only one who can get better results. That also gives the other person the freedom to avoid embarrassment, without the shame attached to looking foolish or spacey. They're free to give you back the correct information. If you're in agreement, then state the intended promise of action in a summary.

Think of something you want to communicate. Perhaps you'd like the dishwasher emptied before 9:00 p.m. Write down the stages of communication that form a loop.

1. Your request:

_____

2. Your check-in (what did you hear me say?):

_____

3. Promise/contract. Great, so I can count on you for:

_____

Clairvoyant Exercise 4
What If?

What if you were five or six years old again? Notice how

ready children are to share their thoughts and beliefs. They expect you to want to listen, expect you to understand. Who are you communicating with that you don't really expect will want to listen to you? What can you do about it? Ask what if:

I told my coworker/assistant exactly what I need in specific terms

---

I told my husband/wife/mother exactly how this affects me

I explained why this is the way I must do something

A bell went off every time someone really understood my message.

I asked for feedback to make sure my wishes/feelings were known

---

Clairvoyant Exercise 5
Say it with Feeling.

When you're working on communicating tough topics, especially with family members or a team, try making a collage/drawing. Start with words like fairness, loyalty, respect, trust, integrity, and truth. Have everyone create a piece of art around these topics. The pictures should depict people implementing these qualities. Stick figures are fine.

Fairness, Loyalty, Respect: Then have everyone tell what their picture means and what those words represent to them. This can be a great way to open up discussion and reveal meanings you thought were accepted by everyone, but you may find pertain only to the universe between your ears.

Clairvoyant Exercise 6
I Told You So.

List all of the things you think people *should* know without being told. Now decide if you're getting the results you want; that is, are the people in your life aware of the things you think they should automatically know? If so, then you have a working relationship with those people.

If not, you may need to reassess how you're communicating your core expectations. For example: your husband should know to get you flowers for your birthday. Your children should know, your neighbor should know, your secretary, boss, travel agent, etc.

1. _____

2. _____

3. _____

4. _____

5. _____

Your assumptions are correct if you always get what you want—as in our example, you always get flowers on your birthday. If, however, this is an annual battle, then there's work to be done. You must tell him before your birthday that this is an expectation. Let him know the significance you put on it. Ask him if you can count on him for flowers. If he says *yes*, then wait and see. If he forgets again, then you know he doesn't place importance on what's important to you.

So what? If he has a problem with the request, then buy your own flowers. Buy orchids and roses and gardenias. Fill up the house and send him the bill with a thank-you note. Just because you're clear doesn't mean you'll always get your way. What it does accomplish is giving you options to get what you want without waiting your whole life.

When you need a fresh idea, you need to force your right brain into action and then let it visit the left side with new insight. These exercises help you grab a right brain picture and relate it to your current challenges.

Clairvoyant Exercise 7
That's just like:

Using comparison/analogy language uses the right brain. It's a technique that forces you out of the box. When you come to an *impasse* with someone over your expectations versus theirs, together ask these way out questions. Believe us, we thought these were pretty silly when we first saw them, but after we tried it, we got hooked. They also help you lighten up a bit, which is the first step to creative problem solving.

1. How is this situation like a watermelon?

_____

2. Why is this problem like going to the moon?

_____

3. Who in history should play our parts?

_____

Sally

Back in my early days of stand-up comedy I frequented a club on Bleaker Street in Greenwich Village. A young comedian was often there on Friday nights. She was feisty, determined and assertive. Her humor was edgy and told the truth. What was so funny is she said out loud what others of us were thinking, but never said. She busted Clairvoyant in pieces. Her name? Brett Butler. She went on to star in Grace Under Fire. *Many of us remember the classic scene when she is brought into the principal's office for her child who was misbehaving, and the principal said something like, "Well, we can understand the behavior because your child comes from a broken home." As I recall her line was: "It was broken, but I divorced my alcoholic husband and now it's fixed." Go Brett!*

Clairvoyant Exercise 8

Often a miscommunication escalates because we attach feelings that the other person is disrespecting us or ignoring us or in some way telling us that our concerns aren't important. Often, however, we're simply coming from different angles. With both people protecting themselves, it's hard to get past the emotions to the issue. Reframing a concern often gives both people a chance to be objective long enough to deal with the core discussion at hand.

These questions are a right-brain exercise used to bring humor and insight into a problem:

What smells are associated with this problem? (Roses, garbage?)

Name your problem. For example: Jasmine, Running Clock or Runs-with-the-Turtles. Tell why that name suits the problem.

_____

_____

Now rename the project for what it should be, for example: "Mighty Good Gold."

_____

_____

Describe a ceremony needed to set your project in the right direction. How do you get from "Runs with the Turtles" to "Wildfire?"

_____

_____

Clairvoyant Exercise 9

We often think our own point of view is so precious it must be told in great detail. Try cutting out the adjectives and just get to the point. This will always help the people you're talking to understand what you need. If they can't read your mind, at least make your communication easy to understand. Pretend you're on a ski lift, and just as you're about to exit the lift, someone asks you to describe your current job situation. You have six seconds or about twenty-five words:

_____

_____

_____

Clairvoyant Exercise 10

Sometimes we can't imagine doing things another way. We can't imagine having to explain the obvious to others. Now it's time to take a chance. What if there was a way to have your true desire, but in another form. Would you be willing to listen to new ideas?

1. Describe your problem or situation and then come up with the most ridiculous, bizarre solution you can. Discuss what part of that is possible right now.
Example: *An alien queen gives me one hundred thousand dollars to buy a house. But wait, maybe I can get three friends together and form a real estate partnership.*

_____

_____

2. Create a solution to your problem that breaks one natural law and two civil laws. Now what part of this is possible within the law?

_____

_____

3. Name five things you want to feel and two things you want to have regarding your situation. Could you have these things in a different situation, job, relationship, or friendship, etc.? Example: If you're unhappy with your church, could you attend a small Bible study instead for a while?

_____

_____

Reminders

Broaden Your Horizons.

All smart and successful people have a team of supporters. Who are yours? We often surround ourselves with people who think the same way we do. Maybe you need a completely different outlook to jump-start your creativity. If you're a Republican, ask a Democrat. If you're a Baptist ask an atheist. If you're married, ask someone who's single. No matter what the problem area, wherever you assume people will disagree, ask for their perspective. You may be surprised to see how many different "right" answers there are out there.

Remember, if you ask for someone to critique your work, listen without rebuttal. Then always remember to keep the best and lose the rest.

Same Planet, Different Worlds.

People go about their day with various tapes playing in their heads. When you talk to someone, work with them or take trips with them, you may be experiencing many of the same stimuli, but it is being interpreted differently. You cannot expect people around you to be seeing the world the same way you do. In fact, if people ever know what you're thinking, it's the exception to the rule.

Your Action Plan

Remember these formulas when asking for what you need:

☞ I think (here is the situation and my expectations):

☞ I feel (hurt, sad, left out, disrespected):

☞ I want (be specific and very clear in your needs):

Now try this on something you're not getting from the people in your life. For example: help around the house, consideration if you're trying to read, support for your dreams.

Learn to *ask*. We've mentioned some of these "magic" formulas before, but now it's time to practice them!

✓ I think: _____

✓ I feel: _____

✓ I want: _____

Summary

Clairvoyant wants you to spend all your energy being offended because the world doesn't understand you, loved ones never anticipate your needs and you shouldn't have to explain yourself. There's a popular self-help book called *Men are from Mars, Women are from Venus,* by John Gray. In this book Mr. Gray explains that miscommunication between the sexes is because their perceptions of how the world works are galaxies apart. In truth, because we all communicate so differently, we might as well *all* be from our own individual planets. Yet here we are on Earth, looking basically the same, using the same vocabulary, and much of the time meaning something different.

It's time to REVEAL Clairvoyant's awful Lie and realize we have no basis in reality to assume that other people will know what we want, even if we've told them a hundred times. More than likely they're giving us exactly what they think we mean, which is very different from what we actually want.

Now it's time to ACT. Every time you're annoyed because someone didn't read your mind or anticipate a need, ask them how they saw it. While it may seem tedious and time-consuming, the rewards are immense. If you expect that you may have to explain yourself the way you would if you were speaking another language, then you'll begin to get RESULTS. Those results will save time in the long run and greatly limit your disappointments.

To beat Clairvoyant, be willing to ask precisely for what you need. Check to see if you've communicated that clearly. We're not saying this means you'll always get flowers or your children will pick up their rooms every time. But you'll be very sure your needs and expectations have been understood, and that's a powerful way to communicate.

CHAPTER TWELVE
The Monster Lie Assumption

The truth Assumption doesn't want you to know:
If you jump to conclusions, you'll fall on your face!

W e're going to REVEAL how Assumption beguiles you into assuming you know what people are thinking, what people are going to say and what to expect in every situation. In fact, if you listen to Assumption, you often miss great opportunities because you're not even aware they exist.

How do you take control of this Monster? You ACT from first-hand knowledge, not from the biases that often taint our judgment. We'll show you how—by ignoring Assumption, by not labeling people and events based on preconceived judgments—you can immediately improve your people skills, and problem solve with far greater RESULTS. The less you assume, the faster you'll reach your goals.

Meet the Monster Assumption

This is the Monster that leads you to believe you already know everything about someone or about a situation. You use the facts, as you see them. Your own experience is the sole authority on which to base your judgments. Never mind that you might have incomplete facts, or old information, or you may have misunderstood something, or your source was wrong in the first place. Assumption wants you to barge full steam ahead accusing people of things they didn't necessarily do, or assuming things are worse than they are. It doesn't want you to gather more facts or ask for better information, just go on your first and only impression.

The very clever thing about Assumption is that It blinds you to new ideas and evidence. Assumption wants you to be so sure you're right about a certain belief you'll miss all the evidence that could show you another piece of the truth. In this day and age we have to make so many split-second decisions, we don't have a lot of extra time to evaluate all the facts thoroughly.

When people rode in buggies, there was a lot of time to decide which way to turn at the fork up ahead. You watched the turn coming for a long, long time. In cars going eighty miles an hour, things come up pretty quickly. In this fast-paced society, we don't always have the luxury of paying attention to details. We often make snap decisions based on limited information, and then we have to make do with the consequences. It's so easy to base our decisions on assumptions such as: my politics are better; he's stupid; she's arrogant; they're dull; the boss is always wrong.

Assumption's Voice

Assumptions can make us act irrationally, or sometimes can make us appear just plain stupid. Listen to the arrogance in Assumption's deep, baritone voice; each word clipped for effect, emphasizing just how important each sentence really is:

I already know what you're going to do before you do it.

That guy is always a jerk.
This is the best way to do this.
I know what the customer wants . . . the heck with research.
I have a "problem child."
All professors act that way.
You can't please that man; he's a perfectionist.
All men, all women, all people from that place are . . . .

Assumption Exercise 1

Okay, what Lies does Assumption tell you?

1._____

2._____

3._____

4._____

Visualizing Assumption

Assumption looks like a big slug. It is the size of a small cow with a toothy grin that can go from goofy to menacing within a moment. Assumption's bulbous eyes are set far apart on his slimy body. Despite Its shape and bulk, Assumption quickly jumps to conclusions with a fraction of evidence. You would not want to get too close to Assumption because It is a bottom-feeding scavenger.

How Does Assumption Limit You?

When you assume, you close out other possibilities. These

possibilities offer limitless alternatives, solutions and shortcuts to success. The problem is that we get caught up with our own definitions of how things are *supposed* to be, so we assume our way is the way everyone experiences life.

One way to get in trouble with assumptions is to believe that life is going to go a certain way. We work very hard at controlling details. When something happens that we didn't plan, it's easy to get bent out of shape. We forget what our goals are, forget to focus on what has worked out in a positive way. We dwell on the past or the perfect picture or the version of what others thought we would become. We wallow in self-pity because things aren't going the way we envisioned. It never occurs to us that there might be an even better alternative available than what we originally planned.

Assumption Exercise 2

Think of a time when you assumed something and you were wrong. Example: You were surprised how good a meal was. You were amazed how well the shoes you bought matched everything in your closet. You had a good time at a party when you thought it would be a dud.

1. _____

2. _____

3. _____

So often we dwell on what didn't work out. The truth is, many things work out better than we planned or assumed they would. It's important to focus on the fact that things don't stay the same, and that every setback is, indeed, a new arrow to point us in the right direction and get our attention.

Facing the Monster: Our Stories

Jennifer

Back when actress Dixie Carter was one of the stars of the hit sit-com Designing Women, *I interviewed her for an article for* MS. Magazine. *Watching her strut her stuff on the show, I was a little intimidated and assumed she would carry some of that behavior over to her own personality. It was a phone interview; she was in Los Angeles, and I was in New York City at the time. I still remember how effectively she put me at ease, enabling me to conduct a much better interview. Amazing how often we look at someone and immediately size them up based on our current information, much of it imagination or someone else's perception.*

Sally

"Everything in my hotel room is missing. I've been robbed!"

My heart sank when I realized the half-finished manuscript for this book was on a computer in my missing suitcase. I tried not to panic. Perhaps the hotel had removed my things thinking I'd missed checkout time. Surely, I thought, they had my things in storage. This couldn't be happening!

I called the front desk and asked where my things were. The front desk person said they'd check and then asked if my things were missing in room 731, why was their caller ID showing that I was calling from room 631. I assured the desk clerk in my most confident voice that I was in room 731 and that the caller ID had made an error.

Okay, so you've guessed what happened. After several house detectives and I walked around, it was discovered that the room I was in was, in fact, room 631. All of my junk was safely spread out all over room 731. I had simply gotten off one floor too early and housekeeping had left the door open to air room 631. I assumed I was in the correct room, so I never noticed the "new" room had different artwork or a different number on the door.

Jennifer

Sometimes it seems I've created a lasting legacy of bad assumptions. It's almost like my sense of direction. One time, when my son Michael and I were driving somewhere together, he asked, "Mom, which way do you think we should go?" Then he shook his head in annoyance with himself and muttered, "Boy, I must be tired if I'm asking you for help with directions." My reputation precedes me. I'm bad with directions because I miss important cues. That goes double for making wrong assumptions.

So every time I go on "instant assumptions mode" I come up a loser, but I'm learning.

There's a story that Dolly Parton was asked if she minded people calling her a dumb blonde. She explained that she created a multimillion-dollar industry, and you couldn't be dumb and do that. Then she laughed and added, "And I know I'm not a real blonde."

Looking at someone and instantly categorizing them according to an image is mighty dangerous. Now I've got a friend who looks very similar to Dolly, and it's so easy to look at her and make a snap judgment. "Another dumb blonde type. Just look at those (faux) leopard skin pants she's wearing and that slinky little blouse." This woman is very, very smart. First impressions can't begin to do her justice.

Assumption Exercise 3

List five people you know very well. Ask them where they'd like to be in ten years. You may be surprised by the answer.

Person:_____

Ten year goal:_____

Person:_____

Ten year goal:_____

Person:_____

Ten year goal:_____

Person:_____

Ten year goal:_____

Person:_____

Ten year goal:_____

Sally

Once I worked at a big company. I went into the president's office to drop off a report and Gloria—his lovely secretary—was putting on her coat. Since it was only 4:30 p.m. I asked her where she was going. Her reply was, "The opera."

Patronizingly, I asked, "Oh, do you have tickets for the opera?"

"No," she said, "I am in the opera."

Talk about an attitude adjustment. In a moment I realized that this highly cultured, highly educated woman was typing so she could run to practice for the opera in the evenings. She spoke four languages, had a trained voice and had been to places around the world I couldn't even pronounce. I was ashamed and amazed all at the same time.

Assumption Exercise 4
Assumption Busters.

One of the best ways to tame the *Monster Lie* Assumption is to learn to challenge your automatic assumptions. In this exercise list several of your negative assumptions and then go out of your way to prove yourself wrong. Build your own evidence list for the positive.

Example: Assumption: *No one is happily married.*
Contrary evidence: *List three couples who are.*

Assumption: _____

Contrary Evidence: _____

Assumption: _____

Contrary Evidence: _____

Assumption: _____

Contrary Evidence: _____

Assumption:	_____
Contrary Evidence:	_____
Assumption:	_____
Contrary Evidence:	_____

Sally

There was a time right after my divorce when I felt particularly sorry for myself. I had this mental image that I was supposed to be a rich housewife somewhere, and I had assumed this was my right and my destiny. I really resented having to get a job. But I went out and got one.

I worked in retirement centers throughout Harlem and the Bronx. That's when I met Haddy. She was a seventy-five year old woman who still worked a few days a week at the center. I asked her about her life. She had seven children from two different fathers. She'd earned her Registered Nurse's degree by going to school at night for ten years.

She said she had three jobs while raising her children. There was her day work, part-time evenings and weekends. She had Sunday afternoons with her children. She remembers when she had enough money to quit her weekend job at sixty, and how happy she was. I was puzzled by her upbeat attitude. I asked her if she wasn't furious she'd been dumped with the kids and forced to work. She just looked at me and smiled. "I guess I always knew it would be up to me." Then she added, "I always thanked God for those jobs. Some people don't even have work!"

I was stunned and humbled. I had taken "not having to work" for granted. It seemed I'd taken the blessing of a job

*for granted, too. By the way, if you have trouble finding ex-
amples, ask other people to help you locate good examples to
prove you wrong. You can always start with your family.
They would probably jump at the chance.*

Jennifer

*When we decided to write our book, launch our compa-
ny and start our presentation work, we gave ourselves a two-
year deadline. This process usually takes people five to ten
years, but we decided that was far too long.*

*So how do you condense time? First of all you realize that
the world is waiting for your service or product. Next you look
at other people who have been successful and you map out what
they did, only you do it in shorter and shorter time spans.*

*Research how this person accomplished his or her goals
and then sit quietly in a restful position with no distractions. If you're in a place with noisy distractions, put on
headphones and listen to ocean sounds. Now let your mind
roll over the various steps. Did this person open up one store
a year? How could you open more? What would be the dan-
gers (staff not trained, leases hard to close in short time)?
How can you shorten that? Can you hire a staff that's already trained in a similar field? Create online interactive
training? Rent space as a sublet? Forget leases and license
what you do to existing companies?*

*Instead of trying to do what someone else did the same
way, only faster, ask to what they owe their success. Create
your own innovative version with your own time frames. The
only healthy assumption to make is that you need more information and mentoring to take what others have called impossible, and make it possible.*

Assumption Exercise 5
Make Plans, Create Hope.

Every time you give up hope, you've assumed you know everything there is to know about the future. You're acting as if you have the sum total of the universe's collective knowledge. How often do we get into a slump because the information at hand—and historical precedent—says what we want is out of our grasp?

Is that so? Well, who died and made you or someone else the ultimate authority? We give up because our minds are too limited to see all the possibilities. Remember, according to research, we only use four percent of our brain power. We only get to see our little chunk of the world and then act with certainty that nothing can budge. But we're wrong on this one. It's a big universe, and there are a tremendous number of options for how to live and what's really available.

Right now ask yourself:

☞ What do I assume is out of my reach and how do I know that? (a job, a relationship, a home, a calling):

_____

☞ What would I need to do or have in order to get this?

_____

☞ Do you need money? What about bartering? How could you create the resources you need?

_____

☞ Do you need information? (Get on the Internet; it's free at most libraries.) Who can help you?

_____

Assumption Exercise 6
Exploring the gold mine.

Don't you dare assume your life has no meaning or purpose, or that you're too old. At a retirement center recently we noticed one gentleman who was commenting on the change in writing style on the TV show *Saturday Night Live*. His analysis: the humor wasn't as clever anymore. He's currently searching for ways to make his own writing more humorous, and he's going on ninety-six! If you're breathing and reading this book, you have potential yet to discover. The miracle of life is that no one can rob you of your own wonderful thoughts or gifts. The downside of this is they will lay dormant until you get busy and utilize them.

Mining for gold.

Name ten things you love to do:

1._____

2._____

3._____

4._____

5._____

6._____

7._____

8._____

9._____

10._____

Then, list three types of jobs you could pursue, using the list from above.

Example: Love animals: Career possibilities:

Work with veterinarians
Work with animal shelters
Work with animal advocates or animal rights groups
Work in a pet shop
*Plan of action: Get involved in animal associations. Ask
    about job possibilities. Be a dog-walker or pet-sitter.*

Now it's your turn!

Assumption Exercise 7
Shaking Free of Time.

We once met a lovely lady who'd just been a guest of the new Ziegfield Theater reopening gala, because she was one of the original Ziegfield Follies girls. She'd traveled all over the world and was now happy to live on a ranch, where she had a lot of time to read and think.

She turned to us and asked what we thought of Time. "Isn't Time simply a measurement that's been created by humans to define the cycles of the planet around the sun?" she asked. "Truly it's not about aging. Aging is a result of failing health and gravity. No. Time is a concept that really acts to hem people in. People judge their success by how much they've accomplished in such and such an amount of time. But life is not about days. It is not really about minutes. All that is made up by someone else and I don't like it." Wise lady!

We examined our relationship with accepted definitions and beliefs about temporal matters. Then we had to admit we were slaves to this thing called Time. Now, that doesn't mean a person is entitled to be late everywhere they go. But it does mean two extraordinary things:

✓ You can stop beating yourself up about not having more of what you need by yesterday. You can relax and let today be a gift in itself because it's really the only time we've got.

✓ Few aspects of your life must be strictly regulated by Time with the possible exceptions of planes, trains or critical jobs.

List all the ways time drives you crazy. Example: picking up and dropping off kids, getting to airports, making connections.

_____

_____

List how you could change your relationship with time. Example: Do fewer things in a day, plan to be at the airport early and read, allow fifteen minutes between appointments.

_____

_____

Create one hour a day just for you and your dreams. If you can't find an hour block by itself, can you put together moments when you exercise? When you cook? Are stopped in traffic or standing in line at the bank? List when you will make an appointment with yourself each day. Write this down and do it!

Assumption Exercise 8
Jiminy Cricket would love this.

Imagine you're ninety—if you're ninety already, imagine you're a hundred. Now, you're reading a book your friends have compiled about you, what they love and admire about you.

What have they said about your life?

What has stood out?

What was your passion/what did you love to do?

What about your willingness to help others, your integrity, your job?

What do you wish they had said?

You can go in and change history right now! Write your life anew, beginning today, the way you want it lived. Who says you can't? Now add to this book a list of things you want to be sure and do in the next ten years. If you're impatient, do a year-by-year list; some long range, some immediate goals. List the character traits you want (such as patience) and go about developing them by practicing every day!

Assumption Exercise 9
Men and Women.

List all your assumptions about how men act:

_____

_____

_____

_____

_____

List your assumptions about how women act:

_____

_____

_____

_____

_____

Approximately how many men have you spent time with in your life?_____

273

How many of the total population of the world would you guess that is?_____

Approximately how many women have you known well in your life?_____

How many of the total population of the world would you guess that is?_____

What is the likelihood that there are other types of men and women in the world?_____

Would you like to be made right or wrong about your assumptions?_____

Assumption Exercise 10

As you close your eyes, think of the color red. Then open your eyes. Look around the room and notice how many things are red. Good. Now without looking around, list here all the things that are brown in the room:

Brown:

_____

_____

It's amazing how easy it is to find red things in the room when you expect to see them. In fact, you may overlook anything in the room that is brown because you were cued to look for red. You've been conditioned to assume certain expectations of yourself and others, and you've assumed people would act in certain ways. In fact, you may not even see when people act differently, because you're so focused on what you expect to see.

Reminders

Let go of your preconceptions!

Assumptions don't just limit our relationships. They limit us in every way. We assume life is going to go a certain way: getting a degree entitles us to certain things; relationships should be certain ways; friends will behave in specific ways and relatives in another. When people don't conform to our assumptions we become frustrated, disappointed and unhappy, and often blame God or ourselves because our predetermined pictures of the world simply don't exist—or don't exist *yet*. But by shattering these assumptions, blowing them out of the water, and assuming only that life will be a series of unique experiences, we're open to whatever comes along.

When we believe the *Monster Lie* Assumption, we take very limited information and project it across the board. We think we have the facts and we don't. But based on that very little information, we proceed to behave in certain ways. We get stuck believing we possess the sum total of the world's knowledge and wisdom. It is as if we're hosting a very small focus group of five people and we decide we can forecast from them the flavor of potato chips the entire world will like. When, in reality, all we can tell is what those five people like.

Yes, You Can.

There are literally hundreds of possibilities. Yet, when we limit our thinking—based on society's assumptions for us— we limit our ability to live a joyous existence. Go within and use your imagination to begin seeing all the other possibilities. Begin to renew all the wonderful things you're becoming, and expect to create this in your life.

Your Action Plan

If you want to overcome Assumption, a good start is to familiarize yourself with different people and different cultures. Here are just a few of the books we recommend:

>*Simple Abundance*, Sarah Ban Breathnach
>*Men are From Mars, Women Are From Venus*, John Gray
>*In a Different Voice*, Carol Gilligan
>*Creative Visualization,* Shakti Gawain
>*Reviving Ophelia*, Mary Pipher

To get a better grasp of other cultures, read great authors such as Pearl S. Buck, Alice Walker, or Amy Tan.

☞ Go to the library and read about a different country every month.

☞ Eat in a restaurant that serves food from a different country (Italian, Chinese, Thai, Japanese, Mexican, French, etc.).

☞ Rent travel movies, read travel magazines.

Practice saying: I haven't been everywhere and I don't know everyone, so I can't be sure.

Summary

If you want extraordinary RESULTS, you have to combat

Assumption's Lies. The best way to do that is to expect positive results every single time. Never be so sure that you know how people and things will turn out. You can be very far off the mark.

We've REVEALED that Assumption wants you to live your life as if you already know the outcome—to limit your view of life and yourself to what you can reasonably expect. The truth is that assumptions bog us down as if we're in a swamp.

It's time to ACT. Look around and see what's possible. Ask a lot of questions. Read books about remarkable people who burst their old image wide open. There are people getting sober, learning to love and finding hope all the time. There are people just like you reaching their dreams and dreaming bigger ones.

If you resist Assumption, you can expand your goals, get more of your dreams and reach out beyond your present reality. If you like to travel, you can start believing the entire world is opened to you and it will be! If you're looking for a new career, or a new life in any capacity, you'll start to see it materialize. In other words, you can dream beyond anything you've dared. By controlling Assumption, you have every chance to achieve those dreams. You just have to start. Take any baby step and keep opening your mind a little more each day

CHAPTER THIRTEEN

The Monster Lie Sandman

The truth Sandman doesn't want you to know:
Sleep is easy. It takes courage to stay awake.

Sandman wants you to zone out on your life. To REVEAL the horrible truth about Sandman is to show you how It lulls you into complacency, convincing you that much of what you're struggling with isn't that important anyway. It's not worth all the hassle. Sandman is the "path of least resistance" Monster. Once you realize that falling asleep on your own needs and dreams is a trap, then you need to ACT immediately. By waking up, by taking action against Sandman, you have the ability to handle challenges from a different perspective to get immediate RESULTS on a day-to-day basis.

Meet the Monster Sandman

Sandman wants to pull the covers up over your hopes and persuade you to take a long nap. It might have worked for Rip Van Winkle, but we don't have a hundred years to waste. Every day is precious, and not to be wasted buying into the Sandman mentality that others will gladly try to foist on you.

Going to sleep on your life is a kind of sleepwalking. Like a zombie, you wander about, not really connecting. You can't feel anything. You stumble around for years of your life in denial, feeling unhappy, unfulfilled, powerless. You don't take a realistic look at your marriage, relationship, degree program or job. You play the victim, one who's already been shot and stuffed.

For example: Have you ever had what can only be labeled as a major lapse in consciousness when it came to the men or women you dated? Some women choose men who're couch potatoes, even though they like to spend every waking moment outdoors. Some bright women have dated men who were deceitful, abusive, unstable and selfish. Why? Why would otherwise intelligent people subject themselves to so much heartache?

The answer is, we fall asleep. We believe the Lie that it's better to go to sleep and pretend everything is fine—or at least tolerable—than to upset anyone. The problem is, we don't get what we want or need. We become so used to living like a zombie from *Night of the Living Dead*, we hardly notice what's happening to us, that life is passing us by. If we don't realize what we're doing—to ourselves and our lives—the pain can kill us. That pain can drive us to numb ourselves so we feel neither the highs nor the lows. We need to begin to wake up and pay attention to life, and everything it has to offer. We can't make better-informed choices if we aren't awake enough to learn from our mistakes and feel our pain. Pain is for a purpose. If a splinter hurts, it's to get our attention—and get the thing out!

Sandman's Voice

Have you been asleep for ten years? If you have, then perhaps you've heard Sandman's raspy, wheezy voice as It whispers in your ear:

If you wait long enough the problem will go away.
If you say something, things will get worse. You'd better be quiet.
Things are too overwhelming to do anything, so don't try.
It's too hard. It takes too long.
You're too weak to deal with the pressure.
Others have it worse, so don't complain.
It's normal not to mention feelings.
Don't ask for what you need. It will hurt someone's feelings.
My intuition is probably wrong. We don't have a problem.
I'm probably blowing things out of proportion.

Are you asleep on your life? Are there things you need, want, like—things you've given up on? Where have you stopped trying: a better sex life, exercise, expressing your true desires, a job you enjoy, staying out of debt, staying sober, staying out of trouble?

Sandman Exercise 1

List the areas you've been letting slide, the places you've been asleep:

1._____

2._____

3._____

4._____

5._____

Visualizing Sandman

Sandman looks like an old cuddly bear. It's so cute and sweet and friendly. It doesn't appear deadly. But Sandman will lure you into a false sense of reality. In fact, It'll convince you to join It in everlasting peace, everlasting sleep, and ultimately everlasting death. Sandman wants you to join It in relinquishing the responsibility of your life—to believe that if you stop trying, life will miraculously take care of itself. It won't.

Sandman is always in pajamas because anytime is sleepy time. It's so cute you may not see how lethal Sandman can be. Imagine driving a car eighty miles an hour and being asleep at the wheel. That's your life if you snuggle up and buy into the Lies as this big ball of pillowy warmth whispers gently in your ear. Sandman is very dangerous. It takes courage to "wake up" to Sandman's Lies.

How Does Sandman Limit You?

Sandman wants you to forget about making a difference. Go ahead . . . buy an extra remote, a bigger boat, more land, whatever will keep you exhausted and out of energy so you won't have to face the future or the past. If you're so busy in the present with busywork, too overwhelmed with guilt and sadness about the past, then you'll be too exhausted to feel any excitement and hope for the future.

Of course, there's always substance abuse for a real "unconscious high." Substances both soothe and control you. They take away your choices and your ambition. It's hard to go back to school, learn the piano, or become successful at anything if you're obsessed by a substance. You'll have no drive or energy to change or to use your God-given gifts.

Very often the people who are warning you to slow down and be realistic and responsible are the ones who've never had the courage to take the risks themselves. They're truly in a rut. They've been asleep so long, they don't have a clue they're sleepwalking. They want to be sure to pass that minimal existence on to you, mostly because they fear they'll be left behind.

Does this make them bad people? Of course not. But it does often make them pathetic people, worthy of compassion, not to be followed down a path of least resistance. More than likely, they never will have what they want. But their rules, their standards should never apply to you and your life. It's time to come alive and live your life to the fullest, most wide-awake level possible.

Now, we aren't advocating that you be a work-a-holic. If you're a non-stop, twenty-hours-a-day-on-the-go person, you're going to burn out. That can be another kind of sleepwalking. We don't want you to do more work. We want you to focus your work on the right things and work smarter.

Some work is avoidance and some is growth. The best way to test what you're up to is to check in with your body. Are you hopeful and cheerful? Or is life a drag? Is all your hard work delayed gratification for an important upcoming goal: a college education, a house, a baby? Or is it a way to insure you'll never get what you want?

Waking up means knowing who you are. It's deciding that even though growth is hard, emotional work, you will stick with it everyday. Yes, it's hard to work two jobs. Yes, it's hard to go to school at night. Yes, it's hard to eat cottage cheese when everybody else is eating ice cream with fudge sauce. You can do it. You can reach your goal if you wake up and use all your awake energy. Otherwise you'll continue walking around in a stupor and complaining that life isn't fair.

Sandman Exercise 2

List five things that you can do under five dollars that would make you giggle today. Example: Call a friend in another state, rent funny videos, sing show tunes out loud, watch baby polar bears at the zoo, etc. This exercise is meant to get you excited about everyday things; to help you find joy in simple things; to help you feel more human again.

1. _____

2. _____

3. _____

4. _____

5. _____

Facing the Monster Sandman: Our Stories

Sally

There are so many examples I have of going to sleep on my life, that it's hard to choose which story to tell. As a child I dreamt of success. I wanted to be a rock star and a movie star. Then when I got old enough to leave home and make my dreams come true, I was so afraid of success I sabotaged every opportunity that came my way. I went into social work, not entertainment. I stopped painting, dancing or any form of self-expression. I stopped being me and then wondered why I was depressed.

Jennifer

We go to sleep on our lives in different ways. When I was young, I wanted to be a journalist. I dreamed of perhaps being a war correspondent or something equally glamorous and exciting. However, when I had a little college under my belt, my husband moved us to a new city. Between the lack of money and raising my son, I had to quit school. I still dreamed of being a journalist, but by then I was totally convinced no one would want me as a reporter, no matter how tiny the publication or how lowly my job might be.

So what did I do? I got a job as a quality-control inspector for a company that manufactured garbage cans. Did I care anything about using a micrometer, or what went into a "perfect" garbage can? You guessed it, absolutely not. But after all, by age twenty-one, I'd already gone fast asleep on my life. I felt lethargic, unhappy, and totally without control. Periodically I'd interview for a writing position, but always in the back of my mind I believed that if they hired me, it was because they just didn't know any better. As soon as they found out my capabilities, or lack of them, I would get sacked.

It took years before I received praise for some of the articles I wrote when I interviewed people such as Orson Welles, Dick Cavett, Ted Kennedy or the magician Doug Henning, who was on Broadway for five years in The Magic Show. Doug told me my article on him was the best anyone had ever written. I won awards for my photography as well. All along, I kept thinking, "Yes, but I don't really have the credentials, so I'm not really as qualified or capable as everyone else."

Phooey on credentials. When we stop buying into others'

beliefs and fears, we get our very own wake-up call on life, and that's thrilling. When someone asks, "What right have you got to do that?" or "What are your credentials?" your job is to smile and keep right on doing what you want and need to be doing. Unless you need to be certified and licensed under the law, the rest of the "rules" are meant to set standards. These are perhaps needed, but should not stop you from pursuing your dream anyway.

Keep in mind no one has a right to lull you or bully you into complacency, and no one has a right to tell you how to live your life. Only you can rule your life, and by staying awake, you'll be open to outrageous and wonderful opportunities that can only come if you're receptive to them.

Sandman Exercise 3

List all of the important parts of your life. Rate how satisfied you are with each one. The areas that are not quite up to par are places you can begin to change for the better today. Want a better job? Get more training. Want a happier marriage? Get counseling to be a happier person.

Life area: *Satisfaction level 1 (low)–5 (high):*

1. Home life _____

2. Work/career _____

3. Health/fitness _____

4. Spiritual life/church _____

5. _____

6._____

7._____

8._____

9._____

10._____

Create a plan to get your life where you want it to be, beginning right now!

Human beings need to express themselves: their joys, their pain, their experiences. If you live where no one will hear you, then you begin to wither and die. Human beings like to use their gifts as a way to express feelings and strengths. If they're denied, they begin to have self-doubt and their self-esteem crashes. They believe they have little or no value.

Jennifer

We go to sleep because we believe the Lie that we can't have our dreams. When the brain kills off enthusiasm, visions, and self-confidence, then the body starts to shut down. Our appetite goes helter-skelter, too little or too much. Our center has melted and we're out of balance. The body falls apart in a last-ditch effort to get some attention. That's why so many people call their first heart attack "The Big Wake-Up Call." Our bodies are alerting us that it's time to wake up, to get past the denial, the "I'll-sleep-through-it" mentality.

Our bodies tell us when we're not in sync, sometime in

small ways like a cold or feeling irritable. Along with sickness and depression, let's not forget being accident-prone. Car accidents, falling accidents, kitchen accidents, boating accidents involve many people who are not in control.

Where are they? Asleep on their lives. Either they're so out of it they miss the warning signals before an accident, or they're in such pain that they're driving themselves to destruction. Either way, the results can be devastating.

If you were to ask all these people if they're ready to die, the response would be an immediate no. But if you ask them—or ask yourself—When did you start dying? When did the process begin? Most people know exactly when it was. It usually centers around some huge disappointment in life. We're so shattered that we close down, and sleep creeps upon us like mildew in the basement. It can happen at age four, fourteen, or forty.

Sandman Exercise 4

It's not a good idea to stop creating and participating in an area that gives you joy, just because someone in your life doesn't appreciate it. Do you decorate cakes? Keep decorating. Do you glue stones together into sculpture? Glue away. Do you garden? Keep digging.

To stop practicing your natural creativity is to deny a stream of exuberance that makes you human. It's like stifling a sneeze. The pressure of withholding can cause you to feel as if your head is exploding. A sure way to kill yourself off while you're still breathing is to deny yourself expression. Part of the process of denial is to give up, give in, quit trying to fight, give away your control.

List three things you used to love to do that you've stopped:

1._____

2._____

3._____

If you stopped for health reasons, is there any part of that activity you can still be involved with? Bad knees? Can't ski? Can you organize ski races for kids? Can't sing and dance on stage? Can you work with the young or the elderly and coach them or direct a musical?

Sandman Exercise 5
Copping an Attitude.

Interview twenty-five very successful people. Research, find truly successful people and get a few minutes of their time. You can tell them you're doing a research project (you are) or find friends of friends and name-drop, or whatever works.

Ask them:

1. How has your attitude affected your success?

_____

2. Do you believe you can create your own reality?

_____

3. How do you maintain this core belief when faced with a blitz of negativity?

_____

4. What steps did they take to create the reality they have in their lives right now?

Then write a four-step formula composed of their answers, and study this for five minutes every morning, at lunch and every night for a month. Watch the results!

Sandman Exercise 6
Take your pulse!

Are you asleep on your life? Ask yourself these questions:

☞ Is your body happy living with you or not? Do you show symptoms of stress, headaches, muscle aches, nausea?

☞ Are you confident you can have your heart's desire? If the sound of that question makes you sad, it's time to wake up.

☞ Do you produce the results you want in your life? Have you lowered all your expectations to avoid disappointment instead of raising them to help you get what you want more quickly?

☞ Are you defensive when others criticize you? People who have self-confidence are not shaken by criticism. After all, you have the power and control, what could you possibly fear?

Sandman Exercise 7:
Rise and Shine.

Before you do this exercise, keep in mind that accelerated learning techniques have continually proven that when you stimulate your creative right-brain, it strengthens your logical left-brain. Pretend you're the most honored and loved queen of a small island. One day, an impostor comes to take your throne and shows everyone false papers. You're then asked to prove you're the true leader of the country.

List what qualities make you eligible to rule this nation:

_____

_____

Now list all the reasons the impostor says you're not fit to rule:

_____

_____

Review the first list. Is it all of the qualities you recognize and hope for? The second list documents all the fears you have of being found out. Could this be the root cause of why you're asleep on your life? Now is the time to take back your kingdom and be victorious.

Sandman Exercise 8
Baby Joys.

If waking up all at once is overwhelming, then wake up in stages. The first thing to do is concentrate on simple pleasures, simple joys and answered prayers. Make a list of all the good things you enjoy: ice cream, flowers, sports, books, letters, children, health, prisms, nature, fishing, animals. Surround yourself with simple pleasures and joys. These could be items that are easy to obtain and guilt-free to enjoy, and cost under five dollars.

Example: *Watching a sunset, singing out loud to show tunes, painting your fingernails, watering the garden.*

Things I love to do that I can do often:

1. _____

2. _____

3. _____

4. _____

5. _____

6. _____

7. _____

8. _____

9. _____

10. _____

Sandman Exercise 9
Play Chicken.

No, don't run out in front of cars. We want you alive and

SALLY FRANZ & JENNIFER WEBB

well and joyous and successful. You know why nobody has a good "Why did the chicken cross the road" joke? Because it's all speculation. Chickens don't usually make it across the road. But dancing chickens live to see another day. When we say "play chicken" we mean that funky little dance they sometimes play at weddings and anniversaries. It may be silly, but it's good exercise. Flap your wings, jump up and down, wiggle your backside and dance in a circle. Put on some upbeat music and make yourself breathe. Breathe and move. The best way to wake up to your life is to feel alive. If you wake up the body enough, you can even wake up the mind. You can laugh, you can even do it in front of a mirror and make all the rude faces and motions you want. Did we mention locking the door and closing the drapes first?

List three videos/CDs/radio stations that you love (*The Big Chill, My Fair Lady, Riding with the King,* Mormon Tabernacle Choir, etc.). Play them often and dance.

1._____

2._____

3._____

Sandman Exercise 10
Make a plan to stay awake.

Only those who are alive get to have accomplishments. But accomplishments are battled for over disappointments. Dead people never have to worry about disappointments— they don't care about anything at all.

There's a ratio you can work with here. Be willing to face four disappointments for every one inkling of success. We used four because some days that seems like a lot. When you want something big and new on the planet it might be more like twenty-to-one. If you're going for a breakthrough, it might be more like two thousand failures to one success.

The motivation to stay awake is that you begin to see your dreams come true. The more you accomplish, the more fun it is to stay awake. Soon, you'll be like a little kid the night before a birthday. It'll be hard to sleep because you'll be anticipating all the neat things that tomorrow brings.

Make a plan: I will identify three things I want in my life that are obtainable within a month. Example: Learn a song, paint a picture, write a poem, organize a desk, rescue a pet.

1._____

2._____

3._____

What price are you willing to pay to have what you want in order to stay awake?

How much pain and disappointment will be too much? It's important to know your breaking point. You must give yourself a reward for enduring the discomfort: an ice cream cone, a bunch of flowers, a ticket to the concert or playoff game or a new book. Always acknowledge your efforts!

Reminder

Check Your Attitude.

Author Charles Swindoll talks about the one thing we have total control over in our lives: our attitude—how we choose to look at everything during our day. Yet, ninety-nine out of a hundred people will tell you they don't have any control over the people or circumstances that comprise their days. They believe that other people make them act in certain ways, i.e. bosses who make them furious, parents who make them annoyed, friends or critics who hurt their feelings.

Mary Kay Ash, founder of Mary Kay Cosmetics (the company includes more than 800,000 independent beauty consultants) was known not only for her positive attitude, but for instilling the importance of that attitude into all the people who represented her cosmetics.

Mind Over Matter.

Viktor Frankl, in his book *Man's Search for Meaning*, tells of the amazing choices he saw in the concentration camp he was in. Men with the same meager amount of food, living under the same horrible conditions, all approximately in the same physical condition, survived or didn't survive based on their attitude. Those who were determined to get back to tell their stories, to search for a loved one—or any reason that caused them to be highly motivated—lived. Others who decided there was no hope and nothing to live for—simply died.

One especially sad story is of a prisoner who dreamed of the release of all the prisoners on a specific day. He was joyous, upbeat, and positive for a month. However, as the day approached and nothing happened, he became more and more despondent. On the day he had dreamed they would be released, it didn't happen. He died rather than face the overwhelming disappointment. Within a few days the prisoners were freed, but his despair had not allowed him to live to see the moment.

We create our own realities. Even if 999 people tell you that's not true, they're simply telling you what they believe, what they understand. The fact is, in every instance, no matter what's happening in life, we get to choose our attitude and how we're going to handle every situation. We all get to hold onto hope if we choose to.

Your Action Plan

☞ Do one thing every day that makes you feel alive: eat ice cream, smell a rose, watch children play, take a brisk walk, sing out loud.

☞ Write about your feelings. What happened in the news this week? How do you feel about that? Be opinionated. Get passionate.

☞ Write a letter or an e-mail to the President about an issue (education, environment, gun control, taxes, pornography).

Topic of letter: _____

☞ Wake up to the world of beauty. Name one thing you can beautify around your house: cut flowers, new tablecloth, a candle, put out a bowl of fruit.

_____

☞ Being grateful is a great way to stay awake. List three people who you need to thank this week: friend, neighbor, relative, mayor, child, past teacher, pastor, rabbi, garbage collector.

1._____

2._____

3._____

☞ List six foods you love that you haven't had in three months, but can still eat:

1._____

2._____

3._____

4._____

5._____

6._____

Summary

If you want to be extraordinary, you have to stay awake. Seems pretty basic, but it's not always that easy. Sandman wants you to cut yourself so much slack, you just keep repeating the same mistakes and ignore warning signs that you're in danger. Once you REVEAL how Sandman has kept you ignoring the areas of growth in your life, you can begin to see how to wake up. The real key is to know when you're falling asleep.

Are you paying attention to the type of friends you have? Are you aware of your diet and drinking habits? Do you remember what you're supposed to be focused on to get your dreams? Do you rationalize that you aren't as bad as some people you know? Or have you started to let your integrity slide?

If you let yourself get sidetracked, you'll get drowsy and bored. If you spend all your energy avoiding growth and trying to forget what is important, then mighty soon you could be living a life of unimportance and meaningless pursuits with a tarnished character. Then you'll suffer from low-level continuous guilt; a sense that something is wrong, but you don't know what it is.

If you want to feel awake and alive, you have to ACT. Take little steps to enjoy life, fulfill your destiny. Start cleaning up your act. Drinking? Join AA. Overweight? Join Weight Watchers. Read, talk to successful people, increase your energy around your goals, make that extra phone call, stay up half an hour later finishing an important letter. Push yourself. Stop rationalizing. Do what you know is right even if you're the only one.

The RESULT is that you'll be excited about your life. You won't have to go to sleep on your life because you won't want to miss one exciting minute. You'll get more rest because you'll put in a full day and really sleep.

Furthermore, you'll find that each minute is precious. Each minute is a gift to grow, learn and give to others. You can't afford to sleep through your life; it goes by far too quickly.

Remember the story of Dr. Jekyll and Mr. Hyde? The good Dr. Jekyll was done in by the sinister Mr. Hyde, not because the evil in Hyde was too powerful, but because Dr. Jekyll denied it was there. He refused to admit that he was capable of being Mr. Hyde, so he went to sleep on the fact that he was out of control.

We must watch out for the attitude "That's really not me, that's someone else." We get into trouble when we go to sleep on our bad behavior and cut ourselves slack. "I was tired. I'm under stress at work. The kids are too noisy." Better to admit, "I acted poorly there. I slipped up there. I haven't written that letter yet!" Come clean with all aspects of ourselves. There's the go-getter Dr. Marvelous in all of us, and some days there is the evil Ms. Hyde who wants to bail on us.

So admit your backsliding as soon as you catch yourself, and dig right in again. Get back on the horse, back on track, and every other cliché you can muster. Stop pretending you're okay. Dr. Jekyll was in big trouble. Don't let your personality split. Stay intact by being honest with yourself. Forgive yourself and start a new day. Otherwise, Sandman will have you asleep and giving into your own version of Ms. Hyde.

CHAPTER FOURTEEN

The Monster Lie Worrywart

The truth Worrywart doesn't want you to know:
Worry never solved a single problem.

Worrywart is a familiar Monster. Ever since we were children we've been encouraged to worry, and we grew up to be very proficient at it. We assume it's part of our culture—doesn't everybody worry about something most of the time? We're going to REVEAL how Worrywart tricks you into believing that worrying is part of every solution, and in the process gets you to waste your valuable time and energy in a pursuit that's useless. We'll show you how to take immediate ACTION against this most deadly of Monsters to problem-solve in more productive ways, and to get RESULTS faster—and without the prerequisite worry attached.

Meet the Monster Worrywart

What if it's not about you? What if things happen, or don't happen because of a lot of factors, none of which are connected to you or your ability to worry?

Worry is an investment in the future you hope won't happen. Isn't worry fun? What if___; then___! You can make yourself sick with worry. You can worry so much you can almost believe you have magical abilities and you can make things come true. Worrywart wants you to daydream worst-case scenarios. Worry the new guy will get your job. Worry your new friend will flirt with your husband. Worry you'll never lose weight. Isn't this fun? And when you worry, you never have to do anything to make life better. You're too busy worrying. Worrywart is superstitious, too. Worrywarts are so sure everything is connected to them, they feel guilty if something happens to someone they don't even know.

Worrywart's Voice

Worrywart is so much a part of our life that sometimes we don't even know we're listening to a *Monster Lie*: Listen to this sniveling, high-pitched voice and you'll hear the warnings we've heard over and over in our heads:

If you don't bring an umbrella it will rain.
Murphy's Law: Whatever can go wrong will go wrong.
There is no such thing as a free lunch.
So little time, so much to worry about.
You can't have it until you've paid your dues.
Start preparing yourself to be disappointed now.
It will never last.
Bad things happen in threes.
What if . . . ?
When good happens can bad be far away?

Worrywart Exercise 1

What do you worry about? Where does Worrywart steal your energy? How can you ensure that you spend your time solving problems, not brooding over situations out of your control? The best way to get more energy for your dreams is to discover where the energy leaks are.

List the things that you spend time worrying about.

1. _____

2. _____

3. _____

4. _____

5. _____

6. _____

7. _____

8. _____

Now just imagine you have an alarm clock in your pocket that will go off every time you start worrying. When you hear the bell you'll say this motto: *Worry never solved anything.* Then you'll breathe slowly, deeply. Make a list of some action you can take about your problem. Do the first step before noon that day. It's one of the only ways to stop Worrywart. Otherwise, you'll spend all day with Worrywart, and that's one day you don't get back.

Visualizing Worrywart

Worrywart looks like someone you might spend time feeling sorry for. It looks like a big beanbag chair with bags under

Its eyes and a frown like a windshield wiper mark on a rainy day. Worrywart is gray and dreary and always has a deep sigh on Its lips.

How Does Worrywart Limit You?

There's no such thing as bad luck, there are many chances for life to get complicated because we live in a fast-paced world. Good luck is another matter. There may be windfalls and lottery tickets for some, but the rest of us will just have to count on our wise choices and perseverance, and create our own terrific luck!

Worrywarts are people who start off trying to troubleshoot problems in advance. It's always good to know what the pitfalls are before you start something. It's good to have a backup plan. But you might consider keeping your eyes up as you walk life's highway. Watching your feet means you might not see the low-hanging branches. So often we spend all our time worrying about what might happen, and no time living in the present.

When you worry, you're concentrating so hard on the negative that you begin to only see negative things. Here's a good rule of thumb: Only spend as much time being concerned about a problem as it takes to brainstorm the solution to lead you to the next step. If you cannot control the outcome—"Possible rain for your family picnic on Saturday"— use your energy on Plan B, C and D just in case.

Let's make some distinctions here. If your doctor has just told you that you have a malignancy and to come in next week for details, it's going to be one long week! You could easily go into cardiac arrest or plan your funeral, because even though you may be able to make plans to handle everything from surgery and insurance to estate planning for someone else, it's another thing to be rational when it concerns your own body.

What's the definition of major surgery? Answer: minor if it's yours, major if it's mine. If you're facing surgery, it might feel natural to worry. You can't help it, to a degree. But what if you try to put your energy toward the things that you *can* control? You can control your diet, exercise, family schedules, communicating to loved ones, prayer groups, and facing your own mortality.

Your worry may turn out to be nothing, or it could be very difficult. But if you suffer angst and complain you *will* lose seven days of your life that you still have. This is a time to call friends, be rational and feel the pain of being scared. Fear is different from worry. Fear is an honest feeling that overwhelms you. Feeling scared is when you list what you do know is a concern versus what you imagine might happen. Deal with the things you can do. Use the energy from "scared" and turn it into action.

Has anyone ever asked you, "If you only had one week to live what would you do?" We've heard people say they'd have a week-long party and invite everyone they ever knew. Some say they'd book tickets to see as much of the world as they could. Do you know what no one ever says? I would worry myself so sick I would die three days early. And yet when we hear bad news, that's exactly how we act. If we were really going to die, we might act differently. But instead, we live in this nether world of "what if" and it keeps us from action.

Then there are the professional Worrywarts. They always see the bleak, the glass half-empty. They're oblivious to the fact that every word they utter creates a negative worldview.

They scorn the optimist as not being realistic. A Worrywart thinks that obsessing on something out of their control can actually sway the universe in some indefinable way. It's as if worry will appease God and change the future. Some people believe if they show "the heavens" that they're really upset, really sorry, really scared, or really terrified, somehow all that energy will produce good results, or at the very least stave off more bad luck. We've never seen it happen.

Worrywart Exercise 2

Name three people who worry most of the time and then describe what it's like to be around them.

Name: _____

How it feels: _____

Name: _____

How it feels: _____

Name: _____

How it feels: _____

These people only need their problem to be magically resolved once every ten years by worry for their cycle of belief in the power of worry to persist. Lab rats learn faster than Worrywarts. There's no way of convincing them things are rarely as bad as they seem. They believe worry helps. But again, we've never seen evidence of it.

Facing the Monster Worrywart: Our Stories

Sally

"Don't put a hat on the bed. It's bad luck."

That was all I needed to hear to make me toss my hat right in the middle of the bed. I have a friend who was a rancher. Farmers and ranchers can be very superstitious and pretty big Worrywarts. What if it doesn't rain? What if it does and doesn't stop? I can understand these things are connected to their livelihood and are completely out of their control. Perhaps they feel that if they can project their Worrywart opinions on the universe, they might be able to sway fate in their favor.

But how do you explain football fans who forget to wear their lucky shirt while watching the playoffs at home and blame themselves for the team losing? Tennis players, golfers, boxers and numerous other sports superstars won't set foot out the door without their lucky charms. Superstition is a strange and fickle god to worship. But it also cripples you emotionally.

Worrywart keeps us from seeing what's possible. Instead of asking, "What more could go wrong?" You could ask, "Where is the silver lining on the storm cloud?" Or "What can I salvage from this situation?" Remember the Phoenix rose right out of the ashes, not across the street or on top of a hill. If your life is in ashes, then you can expect a Phoenix to rise right in the middle of the upset, pain and problem. Learn from the pain and move on; look for something good that can come from the experience. Yes, the lesson, the good, or the new direction pops right out of the middle of the painful part. Don't let anger and bitterness cause you to miss it.

Jennifer

"I'm going to die. I knew it was going to happen. It's been in my genes all along."

These thoughts and others kept echoing in my head as the doctor told me I had breast cancer and needed a radical mastectomy. My mother died of breast cancer, and here I was on a rainy afternoon sitting in a doctor's office hearing the same verdict. To say I was numb or scared or panicked was putting it mildly. But I'd learned enough to know worry never made me healthier, and in fact never made me anything but irrational and unable to formulate an action plan.

When I left the doctor's office, I thought of running home and calling several friends. I knew they'd be compassionate and sympathetic, and I also knew I'd feel just as stressed—maybe more so—as I heard the fear in their voices. Instead, I took myself to dance class where I had to leave my worry at the door of the studio for an hour and a half. When I left class, my mind could rethink what action steps I should take.

Today I'm proud to say that not only did Worrywart not get a hold on me, but I also did not need to have the mastectomy. Succumb to the power of Worrywart, and we react to a situation instead of seeing the multitude of options available.

Sally

Sometimes we worry about what other people think and it ruins our self-esteem. My friend Barbara had been out with a nice man on a first date. She was sure he'd call again as he'd promised to do, because they spent most of the night laughing and talking. But the days dragged into weeks, which dragged into months. She spent a great deal of that time worrying about what happened. Was she too loud, too eager? Did he like taller women? Did he want someone skinnier, more feminine, more like his mother, more like his brother?

Then it happened. They bumped into each other at a party a year later. He came right over to her and apologized for not calling. He'd been shot in the head two days after their date while being mugged and had been in intensive care for several months. Seems he had a few other things on his mind—if you'll excuse the pun.

Jennifer

I've learned to be an expert at not worrying, because that's all I'd be doing otherwise. The other day I had seventy people in a seminar, and there was no sound system for a microphone so they could hear what I was saying. There were no tables, only chairs, so no place to put glasses, paper, pens, etc., and minimal air conditioning. Because it was so hot, they brought fans into the room, which made the acoustics even more dreadful. The day before, I spoke to ninety-plus people in a room so long and narrow they couldn't see me. A riser had to be bought in so I was more than a "radio voice."

I'm convinced it does no good to worry. Of course we plan for what could go wrong and have our contingency plans, but there's a big difference between thinking smarter—what can I do to be prepared, just in case—and starting the day with a litany of all the things that could happen.

Worrywart Exercise 3:
Playing the odds.

People who gamble and win understand the stuff of statistics and percentages. They say things such as "two-to-one he'll never get a good deal on a used car" or "nine times outta ten the doughnuts are stale at that joint."

So make a list of all the things that really worry you that relate to your family or profession. Rate them by the likeliness that they're really going to happen to you. Remember, don't say it's a sure thing that if Aunt Hildy and Aunt Mabel both died of lung cancer you'll die that way. You have to add in the fact they both worked in a steel mill, smoked two packs of cigarettes a day and used to ride their bicycles behind city buses to get a cheap buzz from the exhaust fumes.

<u>What you worry about</u>	<u>Likelihood</u>
	(1% not likely; 100% a sure thing):
1._____	%_____
2._____	%_____
3._____	%_____
4._____	%_____
5._____	%_____

What happens if you defy Worrywart? If every time you're overwhelmed by worry you focus on what you have control over and focus on what you want to happen—on the joyous anticipation of the problem solved—the good that can occur. In case you're thinking that's too much blind optimism for you, let us remind you that the alternative is to worry and stay stuck and get an ulcer. Nothing productive will happen from worry.

You plan, you prepare, then something amazing happens. Your willingness to face your fear turns into action and results! It's like a rodeo. The gate opens and you're on the back of the bucking bronco who was asleep in the stall and just woke up kicking. You can only wait to see what happens, and make corrections as you go along. Yes, there is fear, but when you get past that, there is excitement and success. If you continually worry and choose to dwell on those thoughts as you're taking each step, what you do is actually create what you fear the most. It's all a matter of attitude and perspective, and that's something you can choose!

Sally

The year was 1996, and Judy Collins was again in studios recording a song for a video on the war in Bosnia, with haunting lyrics about "Looking in my mother's eyes" for children who would never see their mothers again. The video helped me raise tens of thousands of dollars for UNICEF. Once again Ms. Collins was the creative force behind my activism. In a life filled with worry and dread and whining, Judy Collins has always been a voice above the crowd for many to follow.

Jennifer

I remember being in San Diego once, reveling in the beauty and splendor of the morning. It was so magnificent, so beautiful, and I was about to return to New York City after one final look at the rugged beauty of the California coastline. So I had my arms extended, my face turned upward to feel the early morning sunshine, and I was inhaling the delicious ocean breeze when—splat! splat!—both arms were covered with pelican droppings.

Did this ruin a fabulous moment? Depends on who you're talking to. My son and his wife laughed so hard they were doubled over and in tears. It took me a couple of minutes to wash all the goo off my arms, but I couldn't help appreciating the humor. It was truly a Mel Brooks moment. The Irish have a saying that bird droppings are good luck. It's worth adopting this perspective, because it could happen to all of us.

All kinds of unexpected things are dropped on us, but we get loads of choices regarding what we do about them. Will I worry about future bombardments from the sky? Nope. Statistically it will probably never happen again. Statistically most of what we worry about will never materialize anyway.

Worrywart Exercise 4

If you grew up in a house with worry, it will seem like the natural way to deal with unpleasantness. You'll have to retrain yourself, and at first it will seem both unnatural and wrong. Not worry? How will people know I care? How will I solve the problem? How will I be prepared just in case? How can I stop worrying even if I wanted to? List a few of the things you worry about, large or small, absurd or realistic.

Worry	*Likelihood of happening to me soon*
Example: *Hit by a bus in a big city.*	*1-10*
Hit by a bus in a small town:	*1-100,000*
1.	

2._____

3._____

4._____

5._____

Worrywart Exercise 5:
Needless worry versus legitimate stress.

If you're worrying about serious issues, such as when your alcoholic spouse is going to hit you again (as he does every time he gets drunk), that is not so much worry as being paralyzed with fear. In these situations, it's necessary to immediately put together a plan of action to protect yourself: i.e. get out, get a restraining order, call a battered women's shelter.

Do you have legitimate concerns that need action? If so list them and brainstorm solutions:

Example: Situation: *Violent, abusive spouse*
Solution: *Call protective services*

Situation:_____

Solution:_____

Situation:_____

Solution:_____

Situation:_____

Solution:_____

Worrywart is more about the mild phobias and fears we have, often based on an assortment of information others have told us, or fears we've projected onto ourselves. With these fears, we sometimes believe there isn't anything we can do to stop them but sit and "pray to the worry gods." While the results aren't deadly, or may not seem important to others, they're very important to us. Choosing to worry can create an impotence that really does stop us from moving forward.

Worrywart Exercise 6
Get a second opinion.

Do you have a rational friend, one with a sense of perspective? You need to talk to someone who's survived enough emotional trauma to know which fears are worth being concerned about, and which ones will probably never materialize. Make a "Worrywart Support List" right now, and put it by the chair you sit in when you worry.

Name of friend   *Phone Number*

1. _____

2. _____

3. _____

4. _____

5. _____

6. _____

Worrywart Exercise7
To Hell and Back Again.

If you're having trouble sorting out things that really need your attention, versus all the worries that turn out to be harmless, then you need to copy this page, blow it up and make a wall chart.

✓ Name your problem: _____

✓ Analyze what you need to do to correct it.

✓ Create steps to rectify the situation.

✓ Monitor the results and make necessary corrections.

✓ Your problem is now solved or at least tolerable, and life goes on.

OR

✓ Do nothing, things get worse, you continue complaining, and end up in serious trouble.

Note: The point of this is not to encourage more worry. It is to help you lighten up and realize that life is about handling the problems we all have. The adventure is not the worry of problems, but in the solving of them.

Worrywart Exercise 8
Make Anti-Worry Plans.

A planning guide to help you overcome the ill effects of the *Monster Lie* Worrywart in your life: Write in lipstick or shaving cream across your bathroom mirror,

☞ *"Who will care about this in fifty years?"*

Worrywart Exercise 9:
Who is the Big Bad Wolf?

Decide to go toe-to-toe with the Worrywart inside your head. Every time you're worried, start writing down what it is you want, what's stopping you and what it is that has you so upset. What are you so afraid of?

Are your kids staying out too late? You can worry, or you can quietly sit down with them and negotiate. Let them know you're a basket case every night at midnight. Ask them to call if they'll be late or buy them pagers. If they're insulted they have to report in, explain that responsible adults communicate their whereabouts. It's called caring. Also remind them it's not about trusting them, it's about not trusting all the wackos in the world. No one is safe in an unsafe place.

Worrywart Exercise 10:
Weaning yourself off worry.

If you can't go off cold turkey, then wean yourself off this bad habit. Record your very own worry log and only allow yourself ten minutes the first week, six minutes the next, three minutes the next (per problem). Then get up, turn on your favorite music and do something constructive. Clean out your closet, water the lawn, clean the grout between the tiles with a cotton swab, wash the dog . . . you get the idea.

Worry: Week One.   **Time allotted: 10 minutes.**

1._____

2._____

3._____

4._____

5._____

Worry: Week Two.   **Time allotted: 6 minutes.**

1._____

2._____

3._____

4._____

5._____

Worry: Week Three.   **Time allotted: 3 minutes.**

1._____

2._____

3._____

4._____

5._____

Reminders

Using Questions Like Poison Darts.

If you conquer your own personal Worrywart, you'll still need to shut out the public voice of Worrywart. Have you ever seen a small child get hurt in public? The Worrywarts will come right up to front and center. Say a child has a bloody nose and is lying down waiting for wet paper towels. The worrier will say, "Oh, you poor child, this is horrible." "You must be scared," and "Look at all that blood, maybe we should call an ambulance!" Needless to say, the kid will turn ashen with fear and have the deer-in-the-headlights stare.

In the same situation those who've been inoculated against Worrywart can actually calm down a situation, and in some cases, lower panic and blood pressure. Try saying, "This isn't so bad. You'll be up in a few minutes and you'll be fine." Your confidence can calm down and reassure the child that he'll be all right. Amazing what a difference you can make. In numerous situations others jump right in to forecast gloom and doom. You come in with an attitude to problem solve and find solutions, without putting half your energy into worry.

Ever been pregnant? Have you ever heard those horror stories? Oh, my sister had triplets, in labor for four days . . . . Who asked them? Have a condition of any kind and some people have to unload their fear wholesale.

Channel Surfing.

When the general public can't wait to share their worries with you, be ready! As a reflex action, immediately tune into another channel. See yourself doing exactly the opposite of what they suggest you worry about. This time, however, keep that image twice as long as the "worried" image, and finally blow it up in your mind until it's the size of a wide screen TV. Imagine yourself eating popcorn, sitting in a cushioned chair and watching this positive image. Continue to do this and eventually your brain will catch on. You'll be reinforcing yourself with some very positive images, and the voices of Worrywart will become less and less significant. If you blink and the worry image pops up, change the channel back to the solution! You could even channel surf several solutions or positive, future scenarios. Remember that it takes time to change your habits, so just be patient as you create this new pattern for thinking and having what you want.

Queen for a Day.

Many problems go away when we throw either time or money at them. When working through a worry, ask yourself what you'd do if you had ten thousand extra dollars, or twenty more years. This helps us see whether we're making a good choice or acting out of worry or fear. We may not have the money or years right now, but we need to make sure we're making good choices based on what's best for us, not following the easy way out.

Your Action Plan

List all of the things your mother worried about:

_____

_____

List all of the things your father worried about:

_____

_____

List all of the things you worry about:

_____

_____

What are you willing to stop worrying about?

_____

What can you do about this issue?

_____

List the date you will start

_____

and the date you hope to solve the issue.

_____

Who can help you overcome this worrisome issue?

_____

Summary

We've REVEALED that Worrywart wants you to use up all your waking hours troubled by a situation, convinced you're powerless to do anything about it. The truth is, you can always do something about it. No one can control your thoughts except you. You have the ability to rethink, reframe and readjust to life's unpleasant turn of events. The question is, will you?

The ACTION you take against Worrywart is to make a plan and make a phone call. Stop being paralyzed by fear of the unknown. The sooner you face head-on the thing you're worrying about and see what you can do, the sooner you'll have the things you deserve. We find that once we stop whimpering and whining we have a lot more energy to be proactive.

But beware. You might find it easier to sit around rocking in a chair and worrying than to discover you have an illness that needs immediate attention, or that your child has a problem and needs special glasses, shoes or therapy. Sitting around is always easier, but it's just not productive—ever! If you face Worrywart, you'll be in control, and that's the first step to dealing with life in a way that makes it fun, rewarding and successful. You have the power to make a real difference in your life, and it all begins with awareness, and the choices you make.

Beginning today, silence one of the loudest Monsters around by listing two things that you worry about. Make a pact with yourself that every time you start thinking about these issues you'll switch your thoughts to something else; the positive opposite of the worry. List what can be done to create a different outcome and find at least five alternative outcomes to the one you just wrote.

Conquering worry takes discipline, energy, understanding and a plan. You're free to use all that wasted energy on things that are much more productive, things that will enable you to let the woman that you are shine through in everything you do. Remember though, you need to start right now, in order to see the RESULTS you want and deserve.

SUMMARY

Our Parting Thoughts

Monster Lies are all around us. These twelve are only the beginning. There are as many Lies as there are hopes and dreams. You can't kill the *Monster Lies*. You can only recognize and outsmart them. Remember, you always have a choice in life. If you hear yourself say:

> Well, that's the way it is, and it can't be changed. *Then that's your choice.*
> He made me so angry. *And it was your decision to respond in anger.*
> I'll never be good at relationships. *If you say so.*
> There's no hope. *Not if you focus on despair.*

Find out who has already obtained what you want, and find out how they got it. Do some research. Keep asking until you know what you need. Most people will be flattered and glad to tell you how they became successful.

You aren't organized? Stop pretending it's everybody else's fault. Either make a plan and follow it through, or hire a professional organizer.

Can't resolve relationship issues? Find out why. Find a great counselor. Talk to people who are happily married after twenty years.

Never on top of your finances? Get a financial counselor, practice fiscal discipline or get a better job.

Out of shape? Join a health club, a diet center, or create an at-home work-out you can adhere to.

Lonely? Volunteer in the community or join clubs.

True courage is facing these *Monster Lies,* and realizing if you don't face them there's a good chance you'll stay in exactly the same place forever. By understanding which *Monster Lies* have been tricking you and facing them down, you'll begin to see results. Is this easy? No way! But anything you have to face has been faced by others before you, and overcome.

We wish you courage, patience and continued pride in all the tiny steps you're taking to get exactly where you want to be. Today is a wonderful day for you to begin your journey. Today, all your energy goes toward the future. Your past is truly history. If you're spiritual, then meditate, or bring it to God or a Higher Power.

Remember, you have choices in everything you do. The only thing that will stop you from living your life the way you want to is if you listen to the collective voice of the *Monster Lies.* You were created for greatness. Why settle for less? You know by now you can stop them, and you've got loads of ideas to help you put them in their place. You can expect them to reappear, but each time they do, you can grab this book and find some great ideas to chase those *Monster Lies* away.

By the way, we reread this book all the time. You'd think if we wrote it we'd be experts by now. Well, we aren't. We fall flat on our faces each time we get an unwelcome visit from a *Monster Lie.* We still get thrown into panic about money. We're still aghast that people don't know what we want before we tell them. We still worry. It's still excruciating to ask for what we want.

But now we know what to do. We call each other up. We reread the lessons. We practice these exercises. We make plans. We take tiny baby action steps in the middle of our fear and pain. And it works! Remember: Courageous people are not people without fear. They're people who have fear and do it anyway!

Today is a perfect day to begin; right now, wherever you are, whatever your circumstances—to have exactly what you want in your life. Remember the words of that courageous leader of social change, Eleanor Roosevelt:

"You must do the thing you cannot do."

You are not alone. There are people out there who're waiting to help you. Right now is the perfect time to begin your own adventure